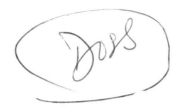

HEADACHE DISORDERS

A Management Guide
For Practitioners

HEADACHE DISORDERS

A Management Guide For Practitioners

ALAN M. RAPOPORT, M.D.

Director and Founder
The New England Center for Headache
Stamford, Connecticut
Assistant Clinical Professor of Neurology
Yale University School of Medicine
New Haven, Connecticut

FRED D. SHEFTELL, M.D.

Director and Founder
The New England Center for Headache
Stamford, Connecticut
Clinical Assistant Professor
Department of Psychiatry
New York Medical College
Valhalla, New York

W.B. SAUNDERS COMPANY

A Division of Harcourt Brace & Company

Philadelphia London Toronto Montreal Sydney Tokyo

W.B. SAUNDERS COMPANY
A Division of Harcourt Brace & Company

The Curtis Center
Independence Square West
Philadelphia, Pennsylvania 19106

Library of Congress Cataloging-in-Publication Data

Rapoport, Alan M.
Headache disorders: a management guide for practitioners /
Alan M. Rapoport, Fred D. Sheftell.

    p. cm.

ISBN 0–7216–4051–6

1. Headache.   I. Sheftell, Fred D.   II. Title.   [DNLM:
   1. Headache.   WL 342 R219p 1996]

RB128.R375   1996   616.8′491—dc20

DNLM/DLC   95–35960

HEADACHE DISORDERS:
A MANAGEMENT GUIDE FOR PRACTITIONERS   ISBN 0–7216–4051–6

Last digit is the print number: 9   8   7   6   5   4   3   2 . 1

Dedicated to the memory of Dr. John Graham, a wonderful teacher, leader, and special human being.

To our headache colleagues around the globe, such as Drs. Lee Kudrow, Jim Lance, and Marcia Wilkinson, who have shown us the way and advanced the science and treatment of headache.

To our wives and children, who have stood behind us and given us the time to make this work possible.

Foreword

The Purpose of This Book

The purpose of this book is to clarify the differential diagnosis and treatment modalities of headache disorders and to validate the very real nature of the pain and disability that accompany them.

Headache is shrouded in myth, and these myths may lead patients to delay seeking appropriate medical care or to self-medicate more or less at random. These myths include:

1. Headaches are all in your mind.
2. Headaches are commonly caused by sinus problems, allergies, hypoglycemia, and temporomandibular joint dysfunction.
3. Migraine is just another word for headache.
4. "You have to learn to live with them."

These destructive "words of common wisdom" are some of the myths that perpetuate inaccurate diagnosis and inappropriate treatment. Patients often need physicians' help in separating myth from fact. And this is in physicians' better interests, too, since informed patients adhere more willingly to treatment regimens.

Too many patients have left physicians' offices with the message that "nothing serious is the matter" and they "have to learn to live with headaches," so they give up hope of appropriate treatment and relief of pain.

One patient told us, "My grandmother lived with headache all of her life; I thought I had to as well."

A doctor reportedly told a 10-year-old girl with childhood migraine, "You'll probably never get rid of them." She left his office in tears. Many patients in our practice come in for their first revisit at 3 weeks into therapy and tell us they are better than they have been in many years.

Our mission is twofold. First, to spread the word that headache is indeed a valid biological disorder that can be debilitating and exact a devastating toll at work, at play, and at home. Second, to emphasize that cost-effective treatment is readily available and easier to achieve than many physicians may think.

We hope that our book will provide the basis for state-of-the-art, compassionate, and highly effective therapy.

Headache in Historical Perspective

> Headache cometh over the desert;
> blowing like the wind,
> flashing like lightning,
> it is loosed above and below;
> it cutteth off him who feareth not his god . . .
> Mesopotamian verse, about 3000 BC

Inextricably part of the human condition, headache has been documented since people have had the means to describe it. Because they were unable to distinguish between external and internal events, the ancients considered headache to be a phenomenon visited upon them by outside forces as punishment for some type of religious transgression. In the quotation above, the reference to lightning might describe migraine aura.

Some of the earliest theories about cause of headache were related to demonic possession, providing a neat explanation for a phenomenon that was otherwise inexplicable. During the pre-Colombian era, trepanation was the treatment of choice. This technique was said to allow evil spirits to exit and was notable for holes that were bored in sufferers' skulls by a copper neurosurgical instrument called a *tumi*. Although our current surgical techniques may not seem as barbaric, many patients nonetheless undergo needless, painful, costly, and sometimes disfiguring procedures. These interventions may include a variety of surgeries related to sinuses, teeth, jaws, sensory nerves, and cervical spine.

Celsus, the Roman physician, described "heterocrania" as follows: "There is much torpor, heaviness of head, anxiety, and weariness. For they flee the light; the darkness soothes their disease; nor can they bear readily to look upon or hear anything disagreeable. . . ." Even centuries ago, the suffering and impact of migraine was described quite accurately; the description is still valid today.

Contents

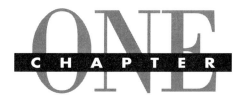

Prevalence and Impact of Headache

Headache Prevalence and Societal Cost

Recent prevalence studies indicate that headache is common and occurs more frequently in women than in men. Linet (1989) reported that 90% of men and 95% of women had one or more headaches in the 12 months prior to one study. She also found that family practitioners are the physicians most frequently consulted for headache problems.

Prevalence studies of migraine in the U.S. population have shown that close to 18% of women and 6% of men suffer from migraine, a ratio of 3:1. This disparity is related primarily to cyclical hormonal changes as well as other factors and will be discussed in Chapter 4.

The Centers for Disease Control and Prevention showed that the prevalence of migraine increased 60% between 1981 and 1989. Whether this represents a true increase in prevalence or is the result of more accurate diagnosis and improved record keeping is unclear. It is evident, however, that headache as a medical condition has an enormous impact on all aspects of daily living. It has a negative effect on quality of life and increases disability at work, at play, and at home.

Many of our patients at the New England Center for Headache tell us that they believe most physicians are unable to appreciate the effect of recurrent headache disorders on the quality of their lives. These patients tell us they wish they could bleed or have a broken bone or an abnormal objective diagnostic test to demonstrate the severity of their disorder to their friends, coworkers, or loved ones. In other words, they suffer for lack of a biological marker that validates their very real but difficult-to-qualify and -quantify complaint.

It is now clear that headache truly represents a hidden epidemic. Headache is the leading cause of absence from work. Approximately 35 million people suffer from migraine, and of these, 79% are employed. It has been estimated that over 150 million workdays are lost each year because of headache. The estimated value of labor lost to migraine is many billions of dollars per year, and productivity losses are profound.

Patients with recurrent headache often feel separated, cut off, and isolated from normal activities of daily living. Migraine affects not only the sufferer but the family and the work place as well. For example, when a patient who is the family's primary caretaker is debilitated by an acute episode of migraine, young children are often put into "parentified" roles, in which they must take responsibility for themselves and for younger siblings. In such situations, the spouse is often called home from work, and frequent emergency room visits may be made. These time-consuming, frustrating, counterproductive disruptions in daily life often have disastrous consequences for both the migraine sufferer (migraineur) and his or her family.

So far as the work place goes, patients often tell us they are very uncomfortable about calling their employer to say they cannot come to work because of a headache. Most people who do not get headaches, including physicians, do not appreciate the intensity of pain, the degree of debility, and the general devastation associated with migraine. Valerie South, the former Executive Director of the Canadian Migraine Foundation sums it up appropriately: "Migraine is not just another word for headache and it is not just another headache . . . it is a debilitating disorder of the central nervous system."

Headache Pain is Real and Significant

Most people who have occasional, garden variety, tension-type headaches ask, "Why not take two aspirins?" This simplistic attitude toward headache leaves migraine sufferers feeling misunderstood, isolated, and even guilty. Many migraineurs secretly wonder if their ability to tolerate pain is considerably less than that of their migraine-free counterparts; they may worry that their headaches are like other people's headaches, but that they cannot deal with the pain as effectively as "normal" people. This negative self-perception lowers migraineurs' self-esteem, which may be frightening to some.

Whereas statistics alone may help us to understand the impact of recurrent headache on patients' lives, they are not sufficient. For example, a Canadian study reviewed the effect of headache on everyday

life and established that migraine sufferers, once they developed some sense of what triggered their headaches, engaged in a significant level of avoidance behavior. Many avoided noisy situations, the sun, and cigarette smoke, and worried about simple activities such as driving. It is important for physicians to understand how those who frequently suffer from headaches often set up an environment that fosters further isolation.

Another way of evaluating the impact of migraine is to examine the phenomenon known as "pre-event worry." For example, women who know that their migraine activity occurs around menses approach that time of the month with great concern, trepidation, and anxiety. When possible, they avoid planning business activities during headache-susceptible periods and tend to become increasingly concerned about routine social events and celebrations. One of our patients said, "You have to guarantee me that I will not have a migraine on October 19th . . . it is the day of my daughter's wedding." Obviously, anticipatory anxiety can have the reverse effect and almost guarantees that a migraine attack will occur. These are but a few of the issues to which caring physicians should be sensitive when they evaluate how patients' headaches affect their everyday lives. A careful headache history should probe for these types of situations.

Self-Medication

OVER-THE-COUNTER VERSUS OFF-THE-SHELF ANALGESICS

Self-medication is the most common headache treatment in the United States. This is not surprising in light of the fact that the great majority of migraine headaches have never been properly diagnosed or adequately treated by a physician. Sixty percent of women and 70% of men with migraine have never been diagnosed and have therefore not received appropriate prescription medication. In the United States, approximately 20,000 tons of salicylates are consumed each year, 16,000 tons of which are taken for headache. This staggering figure does not include the consumption of acetaminophen and ibuprofen.

A section of shelves clearly marked "Headache" (Fig. 1–1) is a fixture in many pharmacies throughout the United States. Here, the space allocated for relief of headache pain may be as long as 30 feet and as high as 6 feet. These shelves hold a wide variety of analgesic, sinus, and allergy medications—all positioned by manufacturers for treatment of headache. Many offerings on these shelves are combination agents that contain various pain relievers, vasoconstrictors, antihistamines, and caffeine.

Historically these have been called over-the-counter medicines. Nowadays, however, the only medication that passes over the counter is prescription medication. Nonprescription medication is not over-the-counter but is in fact off-the-shelf. This distinction is important because over-the-counter medication used to be supervised by pharmacists who might comment to a consumer, for instance, that a current purchase represents the second or third bottle of salicylates bought in the last 2 weeks. Now most purchases are unsupervised. The problem is compounded by the fact that the majority of nonprescription analgesics are not even purchased at pharmacies; they are bought in combination superstores, supermarkets, and convenience stores that do not have pharmacists available to help consumers.

A DETAILED HISTORY IS CRITICAL

Given the preceding tendencies on the part of headache sufferers, it is vital that physicians obtain detailed information about the consumption of medication as part of the headache history. Such information should include all types of medicine—prescription and off-the-shelf—taken, numbers of pills per day or week, and duration of use. Although this type of information is a key factor in making an accurate diagnosis and in mapping appropriate treatment, physicians often do not probe for it.

CONSEQUENCES OF ANALGESIC OVERUSE

Rebound headache, an intensification of severity and prolongation of the headache process, and toxic reaction to medication are among the more serious consequences of the overuse of analgesics and other medications that deliver symptomatic relief of headache pain. Salicylates may be toxic to the eighth cranial nerve, and overuse can result in tinnitus, gastrointestinal bleeding, and easy bruisability. Furthermore, prolonged use of either salicylates or nonsteroidal anti-inflammatory agents can result in kidney damage or stomach pain or both. Acetaminophen taken in excessive amounts over several months has been demonstrated to be hepatotoxic in some cases.

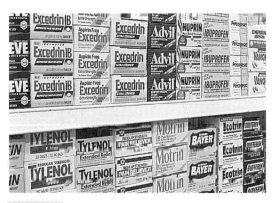

Figure 1–1

Typical off-the-shelf assortment of medications for headache relief at a local pharmacy. Collections like this one can be found in most pharmacies, convenience stores, and department stores. Patients have a wide selection of simple and compound analgesics to choose from and do not need to consult a pharmacist before purchasing medication.

Why Do Consumers Have So Poor An Understanding of Recurrent Headache Disorders?

No off-the-shelf analgesic marketed in the United States is permitted to carry labeling that indicates its utility in relieving migraine headache pain. In Canada and in some European countries, some nonprescription medications are approved for migraine and are labeled as such. Labeling regulations in the United States leave manufacturers running advertisements that tell consumers to take off-the-shelf analgesics for "stress headaches, bad headaches, sinus headaches, and allergy headaches."

The visual message, however, may be in direct contrast to this labeling constraint. A recent television commercial features a woman made completely dysfunctional by pain; she sits in a dark room, holding one side of her head. Her husband is outside the room telling the couple's children that "Mom has another one of her sinus headaches." This type of message may be at least partially responsible for the mistaken belief that headaches are often caused by sinus and allergy problems. This is true only in a small minority of cases, which will be discussed in greater depth in Chapter 3. The vast majority of patients who use nonprescription analgesics and sinus medications are probably overmedicating for migraine, chronic daily headache, chronic tension-type headache, and related disorders.

Consequences of Misdiagnosis and Inappropriate Treatment

The consequences of misdiagnosis and inappropriate treatment include dependency on or addiction to pain killers, repeated and unnecessary testing, hospitalization, frequent emergency room visits, and unnecessary procedures. In addition to these direct costs, indirect or harder-to-quantify costs of mismanagement of headache pain include significant disability, anxiety, depression, dysfunction, and disruption of the family. In short, the deleterious consequences of misdiagnosis and treatment of chronic and severe headache are expensive in both human and financial terms. These costs are of more concern than ever, given rising sensitivity to human values and increasing concerns about health care efficiency and cost of treatment.

With these thoughts in mind, we hope you will find that the following chapters enhance your understanding and management of headache in your daily practice.

SUGGESTED READINGS

Celentano DD, Stewart WF, Lipton RB, et al: Medication use and disability among migraineurs: A national probability sample survey. *Headache.* 1992;32:223.

Division of Health Care Statistics, National Center for Health Statistics, Centers for Disease Control: Illness disability statistics: Division of Health Interview Statistics and National Ambulatory Medical Care Survey. *MMWR.* 1991;40:331.

Linet MS, Stewart WF, Celentano DD, et al: An epidemiologic study of headache among adolescents and young adults. *JAMA.* 1989;261:2211.

Lipton RB: An overview of epidemiology of common primary headaches. *Headache.* 1994;34(Suppl 1):2.

Osterhaus JT, Townsend RJ: The quality of life of migraineurs: A cross sectional profile. *Cephalalgia.* 1991;11(Suppl 11):103.

Pryse-Phillips W, Findlay H, Tuswell P, et al: A Canadian population survey on the clinical, epidemiologic and societal impact of migraine and tension-type headache. *Can J Neurol Sci.* 1992;19:333.

Rapoport AM, Weeks RE, Sheftell FD, et al: Analgesic rebound headache: Theoretical and practical implications. *Cephalalgia.* 1985(Suppl 3):448.

Solomon GD, Skobieranda FA, Gragg LA: Quality of life and well-being of headache patients: Measurement by the medical outcomes study instrument. *Headache.* 1993;33:351.

Solomon S: OTC analgesics in treating common primary headaches: A review of safety and efficacy. *Headache.* 1994(Suppl 1):13.

Stewart WF, Celentano DD, Linet MS: Disability, physician consultation, and use of prescription medication in a population-based study of headache. *Biomed Pharmacother.* 1989;43:711.

Stewart WF, Lipton RB, Celentano DD, et al: The epidemiology of severe migraine headaches from a national survey: Implications of projections to the United States population. *Cephalalgia.* 1991;11 (Suppl 11):87.

Stewart WF, Lipton RB, Celentano DD, et al: Prevalence of migraine headache in the United States. *JAMA.* 1992;267:64.

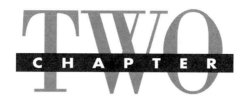

Diagnosis and Classification of Headache Disorders

Now, more than ever before, classification of headache is critical because it helps physicians to accurately diagnose headache disorders. This, in turn, facilitates more specific and effective treatment. Between 1962 and 1988, a classification system created by the Ad Hoc Committee of the National Institute of Neurologic Diseases and Blindness was the standard throughout the world. A newer, more specific classification system, the International Headache Society's "Classification and Diagnostic Criteria for Headache Disorders, Cranial Neuralgia, and Facial Pain" (Table 2–1) is the standard today (hereafter referred to as the *IHS classification*). It was published in the international journal *Cephalalgia* in 1988 and has completely supplanted the older classification. The classification is associated with diagnostic criteria for the various headache syndromes and has been tested by headache specialists around the world. Although not fully acceptable to all specialists, and in spite of the fact that its very complexity ideally suits it to research and makes it somewhat more cumbersome in a clinical setting, this exhaustive and complex system is helping to standardize diagnostic headache criteria throughout the world. In this section we will attempt to simplify the classification system and criteria to enable clinicians to use it more easily in work with headache patients.

A Simplified Classification of Headache

I. Primary Headache Disorders
 A. Migraine
  1. Migraine without aura (common migraine)
  2. Migraine with aura (classic migraine)
 B. Episodic tension-type headache (acute scalp muscle contraction headache)
 C. Chronic tension-type headache (chronic scalp muscle contraction headache)
 D. Cluster headache
  1. Episodic
  2. Chronic
II. Secondary Headache Disorders (Organic Cause of Headache)

Table 2–1

INTERNATIONAL HEADACHE SOCIETY (IHS) CLASSIFICATION OF HEADACHE

1. Migraine
   Migraine without aura
   Migraine with aura
   Ophthalmoplegic migraine
   Retinal migraine
   Childhood periodic syndromes that may be precursors to or associated with migraine
   Complications of migraine
   Migrainous disorder not fulfilling above criteria
2. Tension-type headache
   Episodic tension-type headache
   Chronic tension-type headache
   Tension-type headache not fulfilling above criteria
3. Cluster headache and chronic paroxysmal hemicrania
   Cluster headache
   Chronic paroxysmal hemicrania
   Cluster headache–like disorder not fulfilling above criteria
4. Miscellaneous headaches not associated with structural lesion
   Idiopathic stabbing headache
   External compression headache
   Cold stimulus headache
   Benign cough headache
   Benign exertional headache
   Headache associated with sexual activity
5. Headache associated with head trauma
   Acute posttraumatic headache
   Chronic posttraumatic headache
6. Headache associated with vascular disorders
   Acute ischemic cerebrovascular disorder
   Intracranial hematoma
   Subarachnoid hemorrhage
   Unruptured vascular malformation
   Arteritis
   Carotid or vertebral artery pain
   Venous thrombosis
   Arterial hypertension
   Headache associated with other vascular disorder
7. Headache associated with nonvascular intracranial disorder
   High CSF pressure
   Low CSF pressure
   Intracranial infection
   Intracranial sarcoidosis and other noninfectious inflammatory diseases
   Headache related to intrathecal injections
   Intracranial neoplasm
   Headache associated with other intracranial disorder
8. Headache associated with substances or their withdrawal
   Headache induced by acute substance use or exposure
   Headache induced by chronic substance use or exposure
   Headache from substance withdrawal (acute use)
   Headache from substance withdrawal (chronic use)
   Headache associated with substances but with uncertain mechanism
9. Headache associated with noncephalic infection
   Viral infection
   Bacterial infection
   Headache related to other infection
10. Headache associated with metabolic disorder
    Hypoxia
    Hypercapnia
    Mixed hypoxia and hypercapnia
    Hypoglycemia
    Dialysis
    Headache related to other metabolic abnormality
11. Headache or facial pain associated with disorder of cranium, neck, eyes, ears, nose, sinuses, teeth, mouth, or other facial or cranial structures
    Cranial bone
    Neck
    Eyes
    Ears
    Nose and sinuses
    Teeth, jaws, and related structures
    Temporomandibular joint disease
12. Cranial neuralgias, nerve trunk pain, and deafferentation pain
    Persistent (in contrast to tic-like) pain of cranial nerve origin
    Trigeminal neuralgia
    Glossopharyngeal neuralgia
    Nervus intermedius neuralgia
    Superior laryngeal neuralgia
    Occipital neuralgia
    Central causes of head and facial pain other than tic douloureux
    Facial pain not fulfilling criteria in groups 11 or 12
13. Headache not classifiable

Adapted from The Headache Classification Committee of the International Headache Society: Classification and diagnostic criteria for headache disorders, cranial hemalgias and facial pain. *Cephalalgia.* 1988;8:13–17. Reprinted by permission of the Scandanavian University Press.

A. Headache associated with head trauma

B. Miscellaneous headaches not associated with structural lesion (idiopathic stabbing headache, exertional headache, and coital headache)

C. Headache associated with vascular disorders (hemorrhage, stroke, arteritis)

D. Headache associated with nonvascular intracranial disorders (neoplasm)

E. Headache associated with substances or their withdrawal

F. Headache associated with noncephalic infection (diffuse viral infection)

G. Headache associated with metabolic disorders (hypoxia and hypoglycemia)

H. Headache associated with facial pain and disorder of the cranium, neck, eyes, ears, nose, sinuses, teeth, mouth, and other facial or cranial

structures (temporomandibular joint dysfunction, sinusitis, glaucoma)
I. Cranial neuralgia (trigeminal neuralgia)
J. Nonclassifiable headache

We very carefully explain to our patients that all headaches can be classified as either primary or secondary headache disorders. The *secondary headache disorders* are those that are symptomatic of some underlying condition and are by definition less common causes of recurrent or chronic headaches than are primary headache disorders. Secondary headache disorders include such ominous conditions as space-occupying lesions and hemorrhage, and less ominous ones such as sinus problems, allergies, dental problems, systemic infections, and so on. These less ominous conditions only infrequently underlie headache disorders.

Primary headache disorders, on the other hand, are **not** symptomatic of an underlying problem. They are discrete disorders with their own distinct pathophysiology. We will give a brief discussion of pathophysiology of primary headache disorders in Chapter 4 to help readers understand the theoretical basis for the various therapeutic interventions for primary headache disorders.

The Headache Calendar

Although we will discuss nonpharmacological, behavioral, and educational intervention in the treatment of headache disorders in later chapters, the headache calendar will be discussed here because it is helpful in obtaining a clinical picture of a patient's headache pattern. The resulting "map" of the headache pattern can then be used in classifying headaches, in developing treatment strategies, and in tracking patient progress. The calendar is critical for successful treatment of headache. In addition, we have found that a headache calendar helps greatly in improving patient compliance and headache awareness.

Figure 2–1 shows a blank calendar. We tell patients to write their names, the month, and the year in the appropriate places. We have found it useful to have patients categorize headache intensities as mild (1), moderate (2), or severe (3); this will be covered in greater depth in Chapter 5 on history taking. In this scale, 0 represents no headache on the 4-point pain scale used by many headache specialists throughout the world.

Days of the month appear at the top of the form, divided into morning, afternoon, evening, and sleep time in a vertical column. It is important to note that headaches reported during sleep time mean that patients have been awakened from sleep by headache; this box does not refer to the number of hours spent sleeping. The form also allows patients to note headache intensity using the numbers 1, 2, and 3. When the form is filled out properly, both clinicians and patients can see intensity, frequency, and duration at a glance.

Medications are listed vertically in spaces on the left side of the form. These spaces help patients to make appropriate use of preventive and abortive medication and to set limits on medication. This system will be described in greater detail in later chapters.

The bottom of the calendar features spaces in which to record degree of headache relief, triggers, and menstrual days. Patients list relief on a scale of 0 to 3, from none to complete, and fill in the blank every time an abortive medication is used.

The back of the calendar lists potential trigger factors, which will be discussed elsewhere. Marking menstrual days with an X on days of bleeding helps pinpoint the relationship between hormone fluctuations and headaches and is paramount in working with premenopausal female patients.

We use the calendar described for our migraine, tension-type, and post-traumatic headache patients; we use a slightly different version for our cluster headache patients.

Primary Headache Disorders

MIGRAINE

Migraine without Aura

Migraine without aura was previously called *common migraine*. The diagnostic

The New England Center for Headache

Headache calendar

Name ____________ Month ____________ Year ____________

#1 Mild headache
#2 Moderate headache
#3 Severe headache

	01	02	03	04	05	06	07	08	09	10	11	12	13	14	15	16	17	18	19	20	21	22	23	24	25	26	27	28	29	30	31
Morning																															
Afternoon																															
Evening																															
Sleeptime																															

Medication

____
____
____
____
____
____
____

Relief 0-1-2-3 (0)-None (1)-Slight relief (2)-Moderate relief (3)-Complete relief

Triggers:

Periods:

Figure 2–1

Patient headache calendar from The New England Center for Headache. Patients are asked to track the severity of each headache, medication intake, menstrual cycles, triggering events, and degree of relief from acute care medication on a calendar. The completed calendars are discussed with the patient at each revisit and form the basis for treatment decisions. (© 1991 The New England Center for Headache.)

criteria for migraine without aura are listed here in a simplified fashion and essentially read like a Chinese restaurant menu. Patients must fulfill two of the four characteristics of Group A and one of the two characteristics of Group B. The patient must have experienced at least five previous similar episodes with pain lasting between 4 and 72 hours. In other words, if a patient comes to you with clear-cut symptoms of migraine but no history of previous attacks, the pattern to date does not satisfy criteria for a diagnosis of migraine. In our practice, we conduct appropriate tests to make certain that patients do not have an organic disorder.

Group A: The patient must fulfill two of these four characteristics of migraine without aura:

1. The headache is unilateral in location.
2. The headache is throbbing or pulsating.
3. The pain is moderate to severe and may inhibit or restrict ability to function.
4. The pain is aggravated by routine physical activity such as bending and climbing stairs.

Group B: The patient must fulfill one of these two characteristics of migraine without aura:

1. Presence of nausea **and/or** vomiting.

2. Presence of photophobia **and** phonophobia.

We educate our patients to help them recognize when they have migraine, to enable them to use their abortive medication at the appropriate time, and to ensure that they do not take anti-migraine medication for a severe but nonmigrainous headache. Each patient receives a small card and is directed to check the characteristics as described.

Although aura is not present by definition in migraine without aura, *prodromal symptoms* may precede migraine without aura by as much as 24 hours and sometimes even longer. These symptoms are nonspecific and include changes in level of energy, fatigue, exhilaration; changes in appetite; increased sensitivity to sensory stimuli such as touch, sound, and smell; increased yawning and urination; and fluid retention. We recommend that clinicians ask patients if they experience specific symptoms that warn of an impending migraine attack. The following case illustrates **migraine without aura**.

Case History

SR is a single female who works at a television studio in a large metropolitan area. She presented with a history of headache beginning at age 13, coincident with the onset of menses. Initially, headaches occurred sporadically, one at a time every 2 to 4 months. Then, in her mid-20s, they escalated in frequency to one to two episodes per month. Pain was bilateral and described as a severe squeezing and intense pressure, as though her "head were going to explode." It lasted at least 24 hours.

Her pain started at a mild level and escalated over a 2-hour period. It was not unusual for her to awaken with a headache in full progress. During these episodes, severe debility limited her activities; the pain worsened when she climbed stairs. Associated symptoms included sensitivity to both light and sound. During her attacks, SR retreated to a dark, quiet room and tried to sleep. Sleep often provided better relief than did medications.

Figure 2–2 shows the patient's calendar, detailing two headache episodes that were incapacitating for at least part of the day. One was associated with the beginning of menses, shown by the X marks in the boxes

of the menstrual cycle. In later chapters we will introduce the use of medications and show how they are noted on the calendars.

SR's case vividly illustrates that a headache need not be unilateral or throbbing and associated with nausea and vomiting to be considered migraine. According to IHS criteria, this woman has migraine without aura and requires standard anti-migraine abortive agents, to be described later in Chapter 6.

Migraine with Aura

Migraine with aura was previously called *classic migraine*. As in migraine without aura, previous attacks are essential for diagnosis, and at least two of these are required. Diagnostic criteria are identical to those used for migraine with aura, with the following additions:

A patient must have at least three of the following four characteristics:

A. One or more reversible aura symptoms.
B. Aura symptoms that develop over more than 4 minutes.
C. Aura that does not last more than 60 minutes.
D. Headache follows within 60 minutes of aura termination.

(Note: The aura may precede the headache or begin with it. The presence of aura prior to or during the headache defines migraine with aura.)

The most common auras are: scintillating scotomata; multiple small dots; a homonymous visual disturbance that affects one half of the visual field; a hemisensory disturbance, usually paresthesia or numbness of one half of the body; a hemiparesis or weakness of one half of the body; or dysphasia or communication difficulty.

A common visual aura is the perception of multicolored flashing lights just to one side of the point of fixation that move slowly across the visual field and sometimes significantly obscure vision. These phenomena are referred to as "positive" phenomena. Another common visual aura involves scotomata, or "negative" phenomena. These generally start as a dark or black visual de-

The New England Center for Headache

Headache calendar

#1 Mild headache
#2 Moderate headache
#3 Severe headache

Name _____ Month _____ Year _____

	01	02	03	04	05	06	07	08	09	10	11	12	13	14	15	16	17	18	19	20	21	22	23	24	25	26	27	28	29	30	31
Morning			1	2												3	1														
Afternoon			2	1												3															
Evening			3	1												3															
Sleeptime																															

Medication

Relief 0-1-2-3   (0)-None   (1)-Slight relief   (2)-Moderate relief   (3)-Complete relief

Triggers:

Periods:

(Periods row: X X X X X X)

Figure 2-2

Patient headache calendar demonstrating two migraine attacks, one of which is coexistent with the start of the menstrual cycle and the second of which probably occurs during ovulation.

fect, usually in one but possibly both visual fields. The defect expands and generally obliterates some portion, if not all, of the patient's vision. The two auras can be associated, with the phenomenon being described as a large growing black spot surrounded by shimmering lights. The overall shape of the shimmering lights may be crescentic or zigzag lines, which some have called a "fortification" scotomata. The word *fortification* describes the similarity of this pattern to the outline of a medieval fort. Patients describe the onset of this effect as noticing that they cannot see part of a page or their visual space (Fig. 2–3).

Basilar migraine is a headache preceded by aura symptoms that originate from either the brain stem or both occipital lobes. Typical basilar migraine auras are bilateral visual symptoms, dysarthria, vertigo, tinnitus, diplopia, ataxia, and decreased level of consciousness. These headaches are reported to occur more frequently in teenage and young adult women, but this observation is controversial.

Complications of migraine may include stroke-like symptoms such as hemisensory and hemimotor deficits on presentation. These neurological symptoms persist beyond the occurrence of headache and last for several days to several weeks; they are quite frightening to patients.

Ophthalmoplegic migraine involves a paralysis of the third, fourth, or sixth cranial

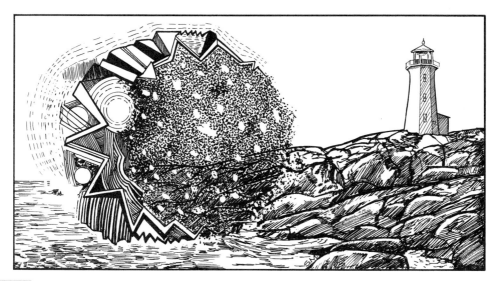

Figure 2-3

Visual aura in the patient's left homonymous visual space prior to the start of an attack of migraine with aura. This visual aura consists of a scotoma with partial obscuration of vision in which there are multiple bright dots and bright-colored shimmering zigzag lines at the periphery associated with geometrical shapes. This aura moves slowly across the visual field and is followed by a severe headache. (© 1991 The New England Center for Headache.)

nerve. The most common presentation is a third nerve paresis, which presents as a dilated pupil on one side, with a ptosis and difficulty in moving that eye up, medially, or down.

Retinal migraine, a rare disorder, presents as sudden onset of a reversible monocular scotoma or blindness of less than 60 minutes' duration. This condition may represent an emergency, as prolonged spasm of the retinal artery can lead to ischemia and blindness, particularly if the episodes are frequent or prolonged. Vasodilators may be required in these circumstances; they help the visual loss but may worsen the ensuing headache.

Some patients may develop an aura without subsequent headache. Some physicians have called this *ocular migraine* or *migraine equivalent.* It is now called *migraine aura without headache.* These patients typically present with the usual types of aura symptoms but no headache. Clinicians should keep in mind that these visual presentations may mimic small tears in the retina; if these occurrences are new, ophthalmologic consultation is necessary. As will be discussed in Chapter 3, carotid artery disease with transient ischemic attack must also be considered and investigated.

The following case illustrates a typical example of **migraine with aura.**

Case History

JS is an 18-year-old male college freshman with a history of headache since childhood. Since the age of 8, he has had attacks four to ten times per year. Episodes typically begin with flickering lights to the right side of his vision. He describes these as multicolored, bright lights in a zigzag pattern that flash on and off while moving slowly across his visual space from right to left. He notices, too, that when he is reading, he cannot see certain parts of the right side of the page.

He also notes slightly slurred speech and that he has difficulty in finding the correct word, although he knows what he wants to say. This effect generally lasts for 20 to 30 minutes and is followed within 10 minutes by a throbbing pain on the left or opposite side of his head from the visual problem. The pain builds in intensity over 60 minutes and is sometimes accompanied by nausea and vomiting. He cannot function for a period of 2 to 3 hours and finds that the pain is increased by any movement of his head or almost any activity. He cannot tolerate light or sound because they intensify his headache. These episodes usually last 8 to 12 hours.

The patient was instructed to place an asterisk on his calendar at the approximate time an aura occurred. Note in Figure 2–4

The New England Center for Headache   * Aura

Headache calendar

#1 Mild headache
#2 Moderate headache
#3 Severe headache

Name _____   Month _____   Year _____

	01 02 03 04 05 06 07 08 09 10 11 12 13 14 15 16 17	18	19 20 21 22 23 24 25 26 27 28 29 30 31
Morning		*	
Afternoon		3	
Evening		3	
Sleeptime		2	

Medication

Imitrex (injection)		1	
_____			
_____			
_____			
_____			
_____			
_____			

Relief 0-1-2-3   (0)-None   (1)-Slight relief   (2)-Moderate relief   (3)-Complete relief

		3	

Triggers:

Periods:

Figure 2–4

Patient calendar showing one severe headache this month preceded by a 20-minute visual aura as denoted by the asterisk. This is an example of migraine with aura. (© 1991 The New England Center for Headache.)

that on the morning of the 18th of the month, he had an aura that was followed by an incapacitating headache.

The case described is fairly typical of migraine with aura; it presents classic characteristics such as unilaterality, throbbing quality, nausea, vomiting, sensitivity to light and sound, and duration of 8 to 12 hours.

Migraine Variants

Several headache subtypes are seen more frequently in migraine patients; these are described as follows.

Exertional Headache. Exertional headache is brought on by coughing, bending, sneezing, straining, exercising, sexual activity, or shaking the head. The pain may last for only a few minutes or persist for several hours. It is often experienced as an intense, throbbing pain located in any part of the head, but more commonly where migraine headache pain occurs. If patients get exertional headaches frequently and with only minor exertion, they cannot usually pursue normal activities and may become disabled. The treatment of choice is indomethacin 25 mg tid with meals if the work-up reveals no serious etiology.

Idiopathic Stabbing Headache ("Ice-Pick" Pains or "Jabs and Jolts"). Migraineurs sometimes experience spontaneous, very brief, sharp and stabbing ice-pick–like pains in various parts of the head. The pain usually lasts for seconds, but it can last for minutes and may occur as frequently as 20 or 30 times per day. Some patients report feeling as though they have been punched in the head; others describe it is an electrical sensation. Patients frequently experience these pains in the area where migraine headache pain occurs. These headaches usually respond to indomethacin.

Chronic Paroxysmal Hemicrania. This is a rare condition that is probably a variant of cluster headache. It occurs more frequently in women than men, an opposite distribution to that of cluster headache. Pain occurs unilaterally, in or around the eye, is very intense and steady, is not usually associated with nausea, and lasts for a brief period, usually only 5 to 10 minutes. Many patients have 10 to 15 attacks per day that often occur hourly with clock-like regularity. Like cluster headaches, attacks are associated with autonomic signs such as a red and tearing eye or a stuffed and running nostril. This type of headache usually responds well to indomethacin and occasionally to calcium channel blockers but typically does not respond to any other form of therapy.

Episodic Paroxysmal Hemicrania. In this unusual variant of chronic paroxysmal hemicrania, a patient experiences paroxysmal hemicrania for several weeks or months followed by a period of no pain. This headache is also treated with indomethacin.

Hemicrania Continua. Some patients develop a syndrome that resembles chronic tension-type headache but is exclusively unilateral. Patients complain of a constant, diffuse, one-sided head pain that is steady, non-throbbing, mild to moderate in intensity, and unrelenting. Sometimes it involves the neck as well. If no other cause is found, the headache is termed *hemicrania continua* and responds to indomethacin 25 mg tid with meals if work-up reveals no serious etiology.

TENSION-TYPE HEADACHE

Tension-type headache was previously called tension headache, muscle contraction

headache, stress headache, or ordinary headache. It is divided into two major categories—episodic tension-type headache and chronic tension-type headache.

Episodic Tension-Type Headache

For a diagnosis of episodic tension-type headache, a patient must report at least 10 previous headache episodes and fewer than 15 headache days per month. Duration of headache pain can be from 30 minutes to 7 days. In addition, the headaches must fulfill two of the following four pain characteristics:

1. Pressing/tightening, must be non-throbbing.
2. Mild to moderate intensity may inhibit but does not prohibit activities.
3. Bilateral location.
4. Not aggravated by routine physical activity.

Both of the following criteria must be fulfilled:
1. No nausea or vomiting.
2. No photophobia **and** phonophobia, but one of the two can be present.

Chronic Tension-Type Headache

Chronic tension-type headache has the same diagnostic criteria as episodic tension-type headache, except that the pain must be present for more than 15 days per month and for at least 6 months. Interestingly, the only other criterion that differentiates chronic from episodic tension-type headache is that although vomiting must not be present, nausea may be. This important issue will be discussed later in this chapter when we explore chronic daily headache and whether or not tension-type headache and migraine are separate or related disorders. Although the IHS classification committee tried to make the diagnostic criteria for migraine and tension-type headache mutually exclusive, gray areas may nonetheless confound the diagnostic picture, with significant implications for therapy and reliability of diagnosis in clinical studies.

The following case represents **episodic tension-type headache**, the most common type of headache that affects more than 90% of the population.

Case History

GW is a 49-year-old female office manager who notes that she has mild to moderate headaches as frequently as three or four times per month, sometimes associated with stress in the office or at home. She describes her typical headache as a bilateral squeezing sensation, which she likens to a tight hat that encircles her skull. At times her headache is bifrontal or occipital and involves the neck. The pain does not throb, and it never affects her ability to function. She is sensitive to neither light nor sound; there is no nausea or vomiting. She may occasionally notice some decrease in her appetite during these times. The pain generally lasts 3 to 4 hours and is usually relieved by the use of simple nonprescription analgesics or even relaxation or change in activity.

Note on GW's calendar in Figure 2–5 that she had three headaches during the month, all of mild or moderate intensity, that were not associated with her menses. Note also that these headaches were self-limited and responded very well to small doses of ibuprofen.

The next case illustrates **chronic tension-type headache**, which we rarely see in its pure form. Rather, it is almost always seen in conjunction with superimposed migraine, as will be discussed.

Case History

SW, a 44-year-old female homemaker, has a history of headache since her early teens. Initially, her headaches were characterized by occasional 4- to 5-hour episodes of mild, bifrontal squeezing pains, which she said were of no consequence and did not interfere with her life. As she grew older, she noted a gradual increase in the frequency of her headaches. During the past 3 years, her headaches have occurred almost daily, with mild to moderate, non-throbbing, aching pain that was bifrontal or generalized around her entire cranium and included the neck. Although these headaches did not interfere with her ability to function, they were nonetheless painful, annoying, and upsetting. She had infrequent headache-free days during the month and denied sensitivity to light or sound, nausea, vomiting, or worsening with exertion. She took simple analgesics on an occasional basis only.

Note on SW's calendar in Figure 2–6 that her headaches are virtually daily, without episodes of incapacitating pain. She takes aspirin only when her headaches are moderately severe and gets reasonable relief from two tablets. She had two moderately severe headaches around the time of her menses. Her history indicated that none of these headaches satisfied the criteria for IHS migraine but did meet those for tension-type headache. Her use of analgesics is within reasonable limits, so there was no reason to suspect analgesic rebound.

Chronic Daily Headache

Now that we have described and discussed migraine with and without aura, and episodic and chronic tension-type headache, it is appropriate to introduce "chronic daily headache." Although not yet an official IHS diagnostic category, many headache specialists use the term and concept in their work. Because patients with chronic daily headache often fail to improve under treatment by primary care physicians, they frequently present at tertiary care headache centers such as The New England Center for Headache.

Chronic daily headache is characterized by generally mild to moderately intense headache on a daily basis with superimposed episodes of migrainous phenomena. It is almost always accompanied by the frequent if not daily use of analgesics or ergotamine tartrate or both.

Chronic daily headache raises an intriguing question: Are migraine and tension-type headache separate and unrelated disorders, or do they represent a continuum that has a common basis within the brain? The following is a typical case presentation of **chronic daily headache**.

The New England Center for Headache

Headache calendar

Name _____ Month _____ Year _____

#1 Mild headache
#2 Moderate headache
#3 Severe headache

	01	02	03	04	05	06	07	08	09	10	11	12	13	14	15	16	17	18	19	20	21	22	23	24	25	26	27	28	29	30	31
Morning																												1			
Afternoon			1																	1								2			
Evening			1																	2								2			
Sleeptime																															

Medication

	01	02	03	04	05	06	07	08	09	10	11	12	13	14	15	16	17	18	19	20	21	22	23	24	25	26	27	28	29	30	31
Ibuprofen 200mg			2																	2								3			
_____																															
_____																															
_____																															
_____																															
_____																															
_____																															

Relief 0-1-2-3   (0)-None   (1)-Slight relief   (2)-Moderate relief   (3)-Complete relief

	01	02	03	04	05	06	07	08	09	10	11	12	13	14	15	16	17	18	19	20	21	22	23	24	25	26	27	28	29	30	31
Relief			3																	3								2			

Triggers:

Periods:

	01	02	03	04	05	06	07	08	09	10	11	12	13	14	15	16	17	18	19	20	21	22	23	24	25	26	27	28	29	30	31
Periods											X	X	X	X																	

Figure 2–5

Patient calendar showing one mild and two moderate tension-type headaches this month unassociated with menses and rapidly responsive to ibuprofen. (© 1991 The New England Center for Headache.)

Case History

AH, a 55-year-old female homemaker and computer programmer, presented with a history of headache since the age of 14. Initially her headaches consisted of debilitating attacks of head pain twice a month, usually associated with menses and ovulation. Attacks would last from 12 to 48 hours and were associated with nausea, vomiting, debilitation, and sensitivity to light and sound.

Her unilateral pain in either the eye or the temple throbbed and worsened with any type of exertion. These headaches were also associated with anorexia, frequent urination, and diarrhea. As she grew older, she noticed a gradual increase in the frequency of her migraine as well as the onset of frequent milder episodes of head pain between migraine attacks. This headache pain was characterized by a dull to moderate, squeezing, non-throbbing pain, bifrontal in distribution, and experienced as a sense of ache or tightness. On some occasions, this milder pain escalated into her more typical episodes of severe, debilitating head pain. She also experienced an increase in disordered sleep and had delayed sleep onset and difficulty in sleep maintenance.

As a result of her chronic headache, she began to experience symptoms of depression as well. Her depressive symptoms included decreased energy, diminished social interest and libido, increased fatigability, and subtle problems in her ability to concentrate that were associated with poor short-term memory.

When initially evaluated, she was taking 6 to 8 extra-strength acetaminophen tablets on a daily basis, sometimes alternating with a mixed butalbital-containing product and nonprescription si-

The New England Center for Headache

Headache calendar

Name _____ Month _____ Year _____

#1 Mild headache
#2 Moderate headache
#3 Severe headache

	01	02	03	04	05	06	07	08	09	10	11	12	13	14	15	16	17	18	19	20	21	22	23	24	25	26	27	28	29	30	31
Morning	1	1	1		1	1	1	2	1	1	1	1	1	1	1	2	1	1		1	1	1	1	2	1			1	2	1	1
Afternoon	1	2	1		1	1	1	2	1	1	1		1	1	1	1	1		1	2	1	1	1	1				1	2	1	1
Evening	1	1	2		1	1	1	1	1	1	1	1	1	1	2	1	1		1	1	1	1	1	1				1	1	1	1
Sleeptime																															

Medication

Aspirin		2	2					4							3	2				2			2						4		

Relief 0-1-2-3 (0)-None (1)-Slight relief (2)-Moderate relief (3)-Complete relief

		2	2					2							2	3				2			2						1		

Triggers:

Periods:

																							X	X	X	X	X				

Figure 2–6

Patient calendar demonstrating almost daily mild headache with eight episodes of moderate headache barely responsive to aspirin. This represents a mild form of chronic tension-type headache. (© 1991 The New England Center for Headache.)

nus medication as well. Although the symptomatic medications provided some temporary relief of her pain, they did not provide long-lasting improvement. Her pain tended to wax and wane throughout the day; it sometimes awakened her at night, and she took additional medication when pain interrupted her sleep.

Over the course of several years, in spite of (and probably because of) her escalating requirement for self-administered pain medication, her headaches appeared to worsen. On one occasion, a physician insisted that she stop all of her medication abruptly, which she did. She then experienced acute rebound symptoms and an intolerable increase in her head pain, which made her debilitated and dysfunctional. She stopped seeing that physician and resumed taking medication.

The patient's calendar in Figure 2–7 shows her daily headache, which varied from mild to incapacitating intensity, and shows daily use of off-the-shelf and prescription medication. Although there were 11 individual days on which pain was incapacitating, these days really represented seven episodes, some of which lasted more than 24 hours. She experienced no relief to moderate relief from her use of medications. At least two episodes of incapacitating pain occurred around the time of her menses. This case illustrates chronic daily headache characterized by chronic tension-type headache, intermittent migraine, and analgesic rebound headache.

Rebound headache caused by chronic overuse of analgesics will be discussed in later chapters. Patients with rebound head-

The New England Center for Headache

Headache calendar

#1 Mild headache
#2 Moderate headache
#3 Severe headache

Name _____   Month _____   Year _____

	01	02	03	04	05	06	07	08	09	10	11	12	13	14	15	16	17	18	19	20	21	22	23	24	25	26	27	28	29	30	31
Morning	2	3	2	1	2	1	1	2	2	3	1	1	2	3	3	2	2	1	3	1	2	2	1	2	3	2	1	2	2	3	2
Afternoon	3	2	2	1	3	2	1	2	3	2	1	2	2	3	2	2	1	2	3	2	2	2	2	2	3	2	2	2	3	2	1
Evening	3	2	2	2	3	2	2	2	3	2	1	2	2	3	2	2	1	3	2	1	2	2	2	2	3	1	2	2	3	2	1
Sleeptime									3											3	2										

Medication

	01	02	03	04	05	06	07	08	09	10	11	12	13	14	15	16	17	18	19	20	21	22	23	24	25	26	27	28	29	30	31
Acetaminophen 500mg	6	4	2		8		2	2	6	4	2	2	2	4	4			6	2			8	8		2		6	4			
Butalbital Combination	3	2			2			4	2			4	2			2	2			2	4			4	2						
Off-the-shelf sinus medication	4	2	2	1	4	2	2	2	6		2	4		6	2	2	2	2	6	1	4	2	2	2	4	2	2	2	6	1	1
_____																															
_____																															
_____																															
_____																															

Relief 0-1-2-3   (0)-None   (1)-Slight relief   (2)-Moderate relief   (3)-Complete relief

	01	02	03	04	05	06	07	08	09	10	11	12	13	14	15	16	17	18	19	20	21	22	23	24	25	26	27	28	29	30	31
Relief	2	2	2	0	0	1	2	0	1	2	3	1	1	0	2	2	1	2	2	2	2	1	1	1	0	0	1	2	2	1	1

Triggers:

Periods:

	01	02	03	04	05	06	07	08	09	10	11	12	13	14	15	16	17	18	19	20	21	22	23	24	25	26	27	28	29	30	31
																				X	X	X	X	X	X						

Figure 2–7

Patient calendar showing moderate to severe headache on a daily basis in a patient who is overusing both off-the-shelf medication, such as acetaminophen and sinus medication, and prescription medication containing butalbital and other substances. This patient has chronic tension-type headache, migraine, and analgesic rebound headache. (© 1991 The New England Center for Headache.)

ache present a therapeutic challenge, from both pharmacological and behavioral standpoints.

Cluster Headache

Among the most painful of all human experiences, cluster headache has often been termed "suicide headache," with some justification. Patients with this disorder have indeed been known to consider suicide if treatment does not help, and a few have attempted it. This headache has also been known as Horton's headache and histamine cephalalgia.

To make the diagnosis of cluster headache, three criteria must be satisfied:

1. At least five previous attacks of severe unilateral, orbital, supraorbital, or temporal pain lasting 15 to 180 minutes without treatment must have occurred.

2. The headache must be associated with at least one of the following signs, which has to be present on the same side as the pain:

Conjunctival injection
Lacrimation
Nasal congestion
Rhinorrhea
Forehead and facial sweating
Miosis

Ptosis
Eyelid edema

3. The frequency of attacks is one to eight per day.

Cluster headache is divided into two major categories, episodic and chronic. Fortunately, the vast majority of sufferers have episodic cluster headache, and only approximately 10% suffer from the chronic form with no significant periods of remission. Episodic cluster patients have cluster periods that generally last from 4 to 12 weeks. The headaches then disappear for an average of 1 or more years, only to return again. Attack cycles often occur at the same time of year, usually in late fall and spring.

Unilaterality is pathognomonic to cluster; only very rarely has bilateral cluster been reported in the literature. Cluster headache pain usually begins on one side of the head and stays there, shifting only rarely to the opposite side during a 2-month cluster period. Patients with cluster pain generally cannot sit or lie still during attacks and must pace or rock, usually with a fist jammed into the eye on the side of the pain. A migraineur lies still and doesn't move his or her head. In contrast to migraine, which occurs more frequently in women than in men, cluster headache occurs primarily in men at a ratio of approximately 5:1.

We can usually identify cluster patients by observation in the waiting room. They tend to be male, slightly taller and thinner than average, are more likely to have hazel eyes, and often have chiseled features, with deep furrows around their foreheads and prominent nasolabial folds. They also present with peau d'orange (orange peel skin) and telangiectasia of the nose and cheeks, and in general have a weather-beaten facial appearance. The late John Graham, MD, of Boston called this a leonine facies (lion-like face).

"Cluster men" tend to be fairly intense and have been described as "macho" types who enjoy outdoor activities such as hunting, fishing, and other sports. They maintain busy schedules and shoulder much responsibility. They are generally very convivial, dynamic, social people who are often heavy smokers. In addition, men with cluster headache tend to drink alcohol to excess except when they are in a cluster period, as alcohol often precipitates a cluster attack within 20 minutes of ingestion.

The following is a typical case of **episodic cluster headache**.

Case History

LK, a 53-year-old white male physician, is tall and thin with hazel eyes, a square chin, and deep facial furrows. He began to experience significant headaches while in his early 40s. His attacks typically began with a burning sensation in the inner canthus of the right eye and right side of the nose. The pain then escalated fairly rapidly, involving the orbit and temple on the right side. He described his pain as non-throbbing and intense and as though a red-hot poker were being thrust forcefully into his eye and twirled. He described the pain as so severe that he has at times felt as though he would like to pluck out the affected eye.

He denies nausea or vomiting associated with these attacks. He reports that his right eyelid droops as the eye becomes red and tears. His wife also noted that the pupil on the side of the attacks becomes smaller than the one on the nonaffected side. The nostril on the same side becomes stuffed at the onset and begins to run as the attack starts to subside. The patient is articulate and describes his attack as a crescendo phenomenon. Typically, these attacks last from 45 minutes to 1 hour. As the cluster period progresses, this patient gets multiple attacks within a 24-hour period and is awakened by at least one attack per night, 1 to 2 hours after onset of sleep. He may have as many as two or three attacks in a given day.

During cluster attacks, this patient cannot sit still or lie down and generally paces with a fist in his eye or rocks frantically while seated in a chair. On occasion, intense physical activity such as pushups may help to alleviate the pain.

Initially this patient's cluster episodes occurred every 2 or 3 years, but for the last 3 years they have occurred annually in October or November. He notes that attacks can be precipitated by ingestion of alcohol and by daytime naps; he travels frequently and has had attacks during airplane flights.

He has consulted a wide variety of physicians over a period of years. Because his attacks tended to occur in the fall, and because episodes were associated with pain around the eye, tearing of the eye, and a stuffed and running nostril, he had been treated by several allergists and ear,

The New England Center for Headache

Cluster headache calendar		
Name	Month	Year
Severity: 1,2,3 1=Mild headache 2=Moderate headache 3=Incapacitating		

Date / Time	1	2	3	4	5	6	7	8	9	10	11	12	13	14	15	16	17	18	19	20	21	22	23	24	25	26	27	28	29	30	31
12 AM			3					3											3									3			
1 AM	3	3		3		3	3			3	3	3		3	3	3	3		3		3	3			3	3			3	3	
2 AM				3								3					3				3	3									
3 AM																															
4 AM																															
5 AM																															
6 AM																															
7 AM																															
8 AM																															
9 AM																															
10 AM								3							3																
11 AM	3	3		3				3		3	3		3	3			3					3									
12 PM					3		3	3										3		3		3	3	3		3			3		
1 PM																											3	3			3
2 PM																															
3 PM																															
4 PM												3																			
5 PM																															
6 PM					3			3												3											
7 PM		3	3			3	3						3	3	3	3				3			3			3					
8 PM			3															3				3	3			3					
9 PM												3																3			3
10 PM																															
11 PM																															

Comments

Medications	Dosage / 1–31
Verapamil 80mg	Dosage: 3 3 3 3 3 3 3 3 3 3 3 3 3 3 3 3 3 3 3 3 3 3 3 3 3 3 3 3 3 3 3
Lithium 300mg	Dosage: 2 2 2 2 2 2 2 2 2 2 2 2 2 2 2 2 2 2 2 2 2 2 2 2 2 2 2 2 2 2 2
O₂ by mask prn	Dosage:
	Dosage:
	Dosage:
	Dosage:
	Dosage:

(0) None   (1) Slight   (2) Moderate   (3) Maximum

Relief	
Triggers	
Periods	

Figure 2–8

This calendar shows a patient having an average of two to three incapacitating but short-lived cluster attacks per day, at least one of which usually awakens him 1 to 2 hours after he falls asleep. He uses oxygen for acute treatment. (© 1991 The New England Center for Headache.)

nose, and throat specialists without consistent or meaningful relief. Oxygen therapy helps.

Although he was found to be allergic to dust and pollen, desensitization and antihistamines did not help. An operative procedure was considered because of a click in the ipsilateral temporomandibular joint, but the patient elected not to have surgery. Since his pain appeared to radiate to a specific tooth, the tooth was extracted, but no relief of headache pain ensued.

As this history demonstrates, typical cluster headache is characterized by periodicity, unilaterality, severe boring oculotemporal pain, partial Horner's syndrome, multiple attacks within 24 hours, and nocturnal preponderance.

For our cluster patients, we modify our headache calendars somewhat to accommodate the phenomenon of multiple attacks within a 24-hour period. It is important for both patients and physicians to understand the rhythm of the disorder, as this will influence therapeutic decisions regarding the timing of medication. The calendar in Figure 2–8 shows that LK's attacks are severe and daily, with as many as three discrete attacks in 24 hours. Note the almost daily nocturnal headaches that usually occur 1 to 2 hours after onset of sleep, often between midnight and 2:00 AM.

It is important, however, not to lose sight of the fact that the attacks of other cluster headache patients may tend to occur toward midday, around noon, and toward the evening. As will be discussed further in Chapter 4, cluster headaches are notorious for their occurrence during let-down periods such as after work.

This brief discussion of the diagnosis of primary headache disorders is introductory to and is intended to provide background for further reading in this book. The information in this chapter will be augmented and put into a more comprehensive context in the chapters on history and examination.

SUGGESTED READINGS

Ad Hoc Committee: Classification of headache. *JAMA.* 1962;179:717.

Edmeads J: Challenges in the diagnosis of acute headache. *Headache.* 1990;30(Suppl 2):537.

Headache Classification Committee of the International Headache Society: Classification and diagnostic criteria for headache disorders, cranial neuralgias and facial pain. *Cephalalgia.* 1988;8(Suppl 7):19.

Iversen HK, Langemark M, Andersson PG, et al: Clinical characteristics of migraine and episodic tension-type headache in relation to old and new diagnostic criteria. *Headache.* 1990;30:514.

Lipton RB, Rapoport AM: Diagnosis of migraine. In Samuels MA, Feske S, Mesulam M, et al (eds): *Office Practice of Neurology.* New York: Churchill Livingstone. In Press.

Rapoport AM, Sheftell FD: *Conquering Headache.* Hamilton, Ontario: Empowering Press, 1995.

Rasmussen BK, Jensen R, Olesen J: A population-based analysis of the diagnostic criteria of the International Headache Society. *Cephalalgia.* 1991;11:129.

Solomon S, Lipton R: Criteria for the diagnosis of migraine in clinical practice. *Headache.* 1991;31:384.

Weeks RE, Rapoport AM: A critical look at reliability of headache diagnosis. *Ann Neurol.* 1987;22:148.

THREE

The Changing Headache, Secondary (Organic) Headache Disorders, and Diagnostic Testing

Dangerous causes of headache are seen infrequently in clinical practice. The overwhelming majority of headache patients have one or a mixture of the primary headache disorders described in Chapter 2. Our goal in this chapter is to help you become familiar with the symptoms and signs that suggest more ominous causes of headache and demand a more aggressive work-up. We will discuss the more commonly occurring dangerous causes of headache, followed by some of the miscellaneous situations in which headache may be a symptom of underlying disease.

A diagnosis of migraine, tension-type, or cluster headache does not protect patients from developing a superimposed, organically based headache at some future time. It is critical to be alert to "red flags" that signal *changing headache* in any patient's history and in the neurological examination. As you work with patients, even your most chronic patients, **always regard the changing headache as though it were presented to you for the first time.**

The Changing Headache

The changing headache presents with different intensity or different characteristics from a patient's usual headache. Changes are subtle or dramatic and must always receive careful attention. The cases that follow provide examples of **ominous changes in headache patterns**.

Case History

LS is a 16-year-old female high school junior who has been under our care for migraine without aura for 1 year. In addition, she had occasional tension-type headache and had been doing very well with dietary modification, biofeedback training, and intermittent oral ergotamine tartrate. Over a period of several months she began to get much more frequent, slightly more intense headaches, in contrast to her occasional, mild, tension-type headache.

When reevaluated by us, she was having a moderately severe headache on and off through-

21

out the day on a daily basis. The pain was diffuse, non-throbbing, and not associated with nausea or vomiting; she also had some difficulty with her vision. For the past year she had been taking tetracycline for acne, and 2 months earlier her physician had raised her dose to a maximal dose for her age.

On visual field testing, the patient was found to have enlarged blind spots, and on ophthalmoscopic examination, what appeared to be very subtle changes of early papilledema. A second neurologist examined her fundi, and in his opinion they were benign. A neuro-ophthalmologist, however, found signs of early papilledema and suggested a lumbar puncture, which showed a markedly elevated spinal fluid pressure (340 mm H_2O).

The patient was diagnosed as having pseudotumor cerebri related to tetracycline overdose. The tetracycline was stopped, and the patient was placed on steroids and acetazolamide (Diamox). Within 1 month her headaches reverted to their original pattern. Without a painstaking repeat history and examination, the diagnosis would not have been made for many more weeks.

Case History

SS was a 48-year-old male truck driver with chronic cluster headache that was well controlled with verapamil and lithium. He came to see us a few times per year for reevaluation and change in medication. Between reevaluation visits, he telephoned to tell us that he had begun to have a different kind of headache. The pain had been building over several weeks and was constant. It differed markedly in quality, location, and timing from his typical cluster headache.

In addition, he was having trouble driving and parking his 18-wheeler. On several occasions, he found himself on the right shoulder of the road, unable to keep his rig in the lane. He was also dizzy, and an ear, nose, and throat surgeon had found no obvious cause for his dizziness.

On examination, the patient had a mild right homonymous hemianopia and made some paraphasic slips when speaking. An emergency computed tomographic (CT) scan revealed a left occipital mass. A search for a primary tumor in this heavy smoker was unproductive until a CT scan of the lungs

was performed and revealed a primary lung tumor. In spite of aggressive therapy, which included removal of both the brain and the lung tumors, SS died after 9 months.

Case History

MA is a 54-year-old female teacher who had chronic daily headache and multiple trigger points for several years. She took antidepressant medication, and on this therapy her headache picture had been relatively stable, consisting of mild daily headaches.

She presented on an emergency basis complaining of an extremely severe, bifrontal headache of 4 days' duration. She had experienced this type of headache occasionally in the past. She improved somewhat after treatment with injections of dihydroergotamine (D.H.E. 45), dexamethasone, and promethazine (Phenergan) for nausea. The next day, however, she arrived at the Greenwich Hospital emergency room with an exacerbation of the headache and evidence of aphasia. An emergency CT scan showed a large avascular mass in the left temporal area. Further work-up that included needle biopsy revealed a sterile brain abscess. This was treated medically with 6 weeks of intravenous antibiotics.

Over the next several weeks, the patient gradually improved and once again has her original mild daily headaches. In retrospect, it would not have been possible to establish the presence of a new type of serious intracerebral pathology responsible for an escalation in headache pain. Only when the patient developed focal neurological signs and underwent a CT scan was the pathology discovered. Patients with chronic primary headaches can develop organic pathology. **Beware the changing headache!**

"RED FLAGS" IN THE HISTORY

1. Abrupt onset of a new type of severe headache.

2. Worst headache the patient ever had.

3. Progressive worsening of headache over a period of days or weeks.

4. Headache precipitated by exertion (exercise, coughing, sneezing, bending over, or sexual excitement).

5. Headache accompanied by generalized illness or fever, nausea, vomiting, or stiff neck.

6. Headache accompanied by neurological symptoms (aphasia, poor coordination, focal weakness or numbness, drowsiness, decrease in higher intellectual functions, change in personality).

If headache pain escalates rapidly and reaches a crescendo within 5 minutes, the headache is more likely to be organic than primary. Subarachnoid hemorrhage is responsible for the most serious type of sudden-onset headache. Other types of intracranial hemorrhage, such as subdural hematoma, epidural hemorrhage, intracerebral hemorrhage, or cerebellar hemorrhage, can all present in a similar manner. In most instances of hemorrhage, patients develop an excruciating headache that is often associated with either a decreased level of consciousness or focal neurological symptoms or signs. Meningitis and encephalitis are less likely to occur as suddenly.

Headaches associated with intense physical or sexual activity can also begin abruptly and may be benign, but they may also be associated with hemorrhage. An extensive evaluation is usually required if severe headache persists and is sufficiently severe that a patient must visit an emergency room. Such an evaluation should include a neurological exam, an emergency CT scan of the head to rule out hemorrhage, and possibly also a lumbar puncture to rule out both hemorrhage and infection. If this abrupt-onset severe headache is not a new type of headache but has occurred in the past and has been fully investigated, then an extensive evaluation is less urgent. However, people with benign headaches can have a *changing headache* and can develop serious organic pathology, as mentioned earlier.

If a patient develops the worst headache he or she has ever had, the pain may have a new etiology. When a patient with migraine or cluster headache comes into the office or emergency room complaining of a headache that is far worse then he or she has had at any time or one that is very different in character from previous headaches, it is important to consider further work-up to rule out organic pathology.

A headache that does not disappear gradually but progressively worsens over days or weeks suggests a space-occupying mass in or on the brain. Most brain tumors do not produce headache until they get fairly large, or unless they are close to pain-sensitive structures. When headaches caused by intracranial masses do become symptomatic, their intensity and location may fluctuate, but the overall intensity of pain progressively worsens. The pain of subacute and chronic subdural hematomas can also worsen over time. Patients with this type of pain should be thoroughly reevaluated, even if they have had negative CT or magnetic resonance imaging (MRI) scans in the past.

When your clinical impression suggests that there may be no organic disease responsible for the headache, it may be appropriate to see if the pain improves with symptomatic treatment only. You should note your plan in the patient's chart. If symptomatic treatment does not bring about improvement relatively quickly, further evaluation is indicated.

Headaches that are precipitated or exacerbated by exertion, such as moderate exercise, coughing, sneezing, sexual excitement, or bending over, can be benign exertional headaches or may be secondary to significant pathology. The brain lesions most likely to cause exercise-induced headache are Arnold-Chiari Type I malformation, third ventricular tumors or cysts, brain tumors, arteriovenous malformations, and hydrocephalus. Whereas benign exertional headache can usually be treated effectively with indomethacin, organic causes must be delineated to match treatment to pathology.

Patients who present with headache associated with fever, nausea, vomiting, or stiff neck may have meningitis or, less frequently, encephalitis. A subarachnoid hemorrhage can cause similar symptoms, so patients must be carefully evaluated neurologically, and a complete blood count, blood and other appropriate cultures, and lumbar puncture should also be performed. In addition, it may be wise to do an emergency CT scan followed by a lumbar puncture to rule out increased intracranial pressure, hemorrhage, or infection.

Although one would expect a patient with

a brain abscess to present with a stiff neck and fever, an abscess often presents only as an avascular cerebral mass without evidence of infection, unless it ruptures.

It is likely that an organic cause of symptoms will be found in patients who present to the emergency room with a headache accompanied by diffuse or focal neurological symptomatology. A thorough history is critically important in establishing etiology of symptoms; further work-up is essential. Possible causes of this syndrome vary from vascular to tumor to infection to demyelinating disease to side-effects of medication.

"RED FLAGS" ON EXAMINATION

1. Abnormal vital signs (increased blood pressure, heart rate, or temperature).
2. Change in higher intellectual functions or cognition.
3. Alteration in level of consciousness.
4. Signs of meningeal irritation.
5. Papilledema.
6. Presence of focal neurological signs (hemiparesis, hemisensory loss, ataxia or aphasia, signs of brain stem dysfunction, or pathological reflexes).

Abnormal findings in the physical and neurological examination are very worrisome in headache patients. Changes in vital signs such as increased blood pressure may suggest an intracerebral hemorrhage. Patients with very high blood pressure are at risk for blood vessel rupture with hemorrhage into the brain. Patients who have had a cerebral hemorrhage, even if their initial pressure was normal, usually develop hypertension. The blood pressure of migraine patients who are in severe pain is often elevated.

A rapid heart rate may be related to cardiac dysfunction, anxiety, or possibly to other medical conditions such as anemia, hyperthyroidism, or altitude sickness, all of which can cause headache. A patient with fever and headache may have a benign condition, such as a viral illness, or a more serious one, such as meningitis, temporal arteritis, infectious mononucleosis, Lyme disease, or any one of a number of febrile

medical conditions that can be associated with headache.

Patients with headache who experience changes in higher intellectual function, cognition, or memory should be suspected of having a space-occupying lesion. Those with psychiatric conditions, Alzheimer's disease, or other types of organic brain syndromes infrequently have headache. Exceptions include hyperparathyroidism and hypothyroidism, as well as carbon monoxide poisoning, which can cause drowsiness, confusion, and headache.

Patients with an altered level of consciousness and severe headache probably have serious organic pathology. They should undergo an emergency CT scan, blood studies, and a lumbar puncture to search for hemorrhage, infection, and tumor cells.

Patients who present with meningeal irritation and headache probably have either meningitis or a subarachnoid hemorrhage. The meningitis may be aseptic; if bacterial, immediate treatment with antibiotics is essential. Left untreated, infectious meningitis can proceed rapidly, culminating in death. Patients with more benign infectious illness, such as infectious mononucleosis and Lyme disease, may also present with meningeal irritation. Patients with human immunodeficiency virus (HIV-positive patients) often develop meningitis.

Patients with cancer can present with meningeal carcinomatosis, which is characterized by headache, stiff neck, meningeal irritation, and multiple cranial nerve palsies. Blood has been found in the subarachnoid space of several patients who underwent lumbar punctures because of suspected meningitis. This finding of blood indicates that the meningitis-like symptoms are due to subarachnoid hemorrhage with meningeal irritation.

Watch for these *meningeal signs:* nuchal rigidity, in which a patient may have difficulty placing the chin on the chest because of pain and stiffness; Kernig's sign, in which a patient complains of back pain when a thigh is flexed onto the abdomen and the leg is extended at the knee; Brudzinski's sign, in which a patient in the supine position with legs straight complains of back pain

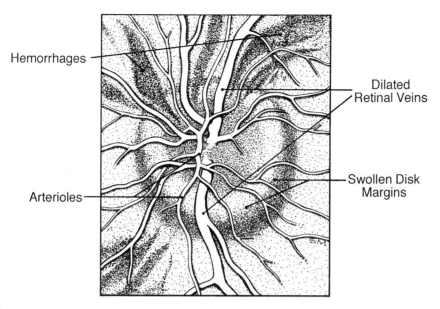

Hemorrhages

Dilated Retinal Veins

Arterioles

Swollen Disk Margins

Figure 3–1

Diagram of a fundus demonstrating the classic findings of papilledema secondary to raised intracranial pressure. The disc margins are swollen, with vessels draping over the edge. The veins are larger in diameter than usual, and flame-shaped hemorrhages are seen off the disc.

when the head is suddenly and forcibly flexed onto the chest; and eyeball tenderness, which is ipsilateral involuntary squinting of facial muscles when gentle pressure is applied to the closed eye.

Any patient presenting with early signs of or full-blown papilledema is a medical emergency (Fig. 3–1). Early signs are slightly dilated veins and loss of venous pulsations (sometimes difficult to see even in a normal patient). There may be some elevation and blurring of the disc margins. Finally, hemorrhages are visible, usually near the disc. These signs are caused by elevated intracranial pressure, which may be the result of an expanding mass or blockage of spinal fluid flow. Papilledema can also be seen in inflammation of the optic nerve as well as in pseudotumor cerebri (benign intracranial hypertension). This latter condition is often seen in young, heavy females and can be induced by a variety of triggers such as tetracycline overuse or excess intake of vitamin A.

Finally, the presence of any focal neurological sign in association with headache strongly suggests intracranial pathology. Patients with these signs should be evaluated aggressively. In some cases, the etiology is

benign and may be a palsy of the third, fourth, or sixth cranial nerve associated with ophthalmoplegic migraine or brain stem dysfunction associated with basilar migraine. In other cases, clinical signs may be caused by what used to be termed *complicated migraine*, a transient neurological dysfunction associated with migraine (as opposed to complications of migraine, such as migrainous infarction, which is a migraine-induced stroke). In this situation, a migrainous aura becomes permanent and persists more than 7 days after the onset of headache. It is, in fact, a completed stroke.

Secondary Headaches (Organic Causes)

INCREASED INTRACRANIAL PRESSURE

Any lesion that raises intracranial pressure is likely to cause a progressively increasing headache. The term *tumor* incorporates any mass lesion (swelling), whether benign or malignant. Brain tumors usually cause focal neurological deficits before they cause headache or signs of increased intracranial pressure. The exceptions are posterior fossa mass lesions, which raise pressure more quickly because the space into which they expand is smaller; they can also block the flow of cerebrospinal fluid. Pain from tumors is usually the result of stretching of blood vessels, especially veins, or pressure on the fifth, seventh, ninth, or tenth cranial nerves or the upper cervical roots. Patients usually complain of progressively worsening headache with nausea and vomiting over a period of many days or weeks. Symptoms of an intracerebral abscess resemble those of a brain tumor; this mass lesion often fails to produce signs of infection (no fever or symptoms of infection and normal cultures, including spinal fluid).

BRAIN TUMOR

The headache from an expanding mass in the brain is usually generalized, but patients may perceive it as localized to the area of the lesion. The pain does not usually fit any pattern; it may be steady or throbbing, mild or severe in intensity, and it usually moves around in location. Its main characteristic is slowly progressive worsening over a period of days, weeks, or months. As such tumors enlarge, patients become nauseated, drowsy, confused, and disoriented and may develop focal neurological symptoms and signs.

TYPES OF INTRACRANIAL HEMATOMA

Collections of blood in various parts of the brain or on top of the brain can produce signs and symptoms similar to those of a brain tumor. An *epidural hematoma* is a collection of blood between the dura and the inner table of the skull and usually follows severe head trauma. An initial loss of consciousness is followed by a lucid period and a progressively downhill course into coma. This condition is more common in children. The pathology is often a skull fracture with rupture of the middle meningeal artery.

A *subdural hematoma* is a collection of blood beneath the dura and is notable for acute findings with rapid degeneration. At the outset, subdural hematomas may pro-

duce only mild symptoms, becoming chronic subdural hematomas over time. Patients with these hematomas present with progressive headache over several days or weeks and some focal neurological symptoms, with fluctuating levels of consciousness. Subdural hematomas may occur spontaneously or with only minor head trauma in elderly patients. Bleeding in these situations is due to rupture of veins that bridge the subdural space.

Intracerebral hematomas are usually sudden in onset and produce incapacitating headache with decreased levels of consciousness and focal neurological symptoms and signs. A *subarachnoid hemorrhage*, often caused by a ruptured aneurysm, produces an explosive, incapacitating headache with nausea, vomiting, and decreased level of consciousness without focal neurological signs. Signs of meningeal irritation and papilledema occur after several hours.

ARTERIOVENOUS MALFORMATION (AVM)

An AVM is a tangle of abnormal blood vessels that may be present anywhere in the cerebrum or posterior fossa. The most common presenting picture is that of cerebral hemorrhage or seizure. AVMs can present as space-occupying masses because they may slowly increase in size. They can be treated in a variety of ways, including conventional or Gamma knife surgery, Bragg peak irradiation, and selective catheterization with the use of small spheres or radioactive particles to plug the vessels. Some AVMs are inoperable; if they present only with seizures, they can be treated conservatively with an effective anticonvulsant.

CEREBRAL ISCHEMIA

Patients may develop severe headaches prior to or during a stroke. Patients with transient ischemic attacks occasionally have headaches. Basilar artery circulation ischemia is more likely to cause headache than anterior circulation cerebral ischemia.

CEREBRAL VEIN AND CAVERNOUS SINUS THROMBOSES

Thrombosis of large sinuses, such as the midline sagittal sinus, or of surface or deep-draining cerebral veins can produce either continuous or intermittent nonspecific headaches. Cavernous sinus thrombosis causes pain in and around the eye, along with a constellation of neurological findings that include dysfunction of the third, fourth, and sixth cranial nerves as well as of the first two divisions of the fifth cranial nerve.

PSEUDOTUMOR CEREBRI (BENIGN INTRACRANIAL HYPERTENSION)

Pseudotumor cerebri has a variety of causes, and patients with this condition present with headache and visual problems along with other signs of increased intracranial pressure, such as double vision with bilateral sixth nerve palsies. It usually occurs in young, obese women and may be related to a variety of conditions and medications, such as endocrine dysfunction or overuse of tetracycline or vitamin A. MRI scans usually reveal very small cerebral ventricles. On examination, patients may have decreased vision, early papilledema, and inability to abduct either eye, which produces diplopia. Diagnosis is usually confirmed by a lumbar puncture that shows increased intracranial pressure. The treatment may include multiple spinal taps to reduce intracranial pressure, weight loss, administration of steroids, and administration of acetazolamide (Diamox), which decreases cerebrospinal fluid (CSF) production.

ACUTE ANGLE CLOSURE GLAUCOMA

When patients present with eye pain associated with periorbital headache, visual disturbances such as seeing halos around lights at night, a steamy quality to the cornea, and nausea and vomiting, intraocular pressure should be checked by tonometry to rule out acute glaucoma, which is a medical emergency.

INTERNAL CAROTID ARTERY DISSECTION

Carotid artery dissection should be considered in patients who present with symptoms and signs that suggest cluster headache with continuous rather than intermittent pain. Pain is usually in the eye or in the frontal area and may also involve the neck. Accompanying symptoms frequently include Horner's syndrome with small pupil and ptosis on the affected side. The diagnosis may be made by conducting a carotid artery Doppler flow study, magnetic resonance angiography (MRA), or carotid angiography. Conservative treatment such as administration of heparin or Coumadin or both is usually indicated and is effective in most cases.

MENINGITIS

Meningitis is an inflammation of the meninges and spinal fluid caused by any type of infection or toxic reaction. It may be aseptic (viral), chemical, or infectious (caused by bacteria, spirochete, or fungus). A constellation of signs and symptoms that include febrile illness, stiff neck, nausea, vomiting, and signs of meningeal irritation usually clinches the diagnosis, which may be confirmed by emergency lumbar puncture and analysis of CSF. Opening pressure should be checked; analysis should include cells, protein, glucose, and a Venereal Disease Research Laboratory (VDRL) test. A culture of CSF should be studied for bacteria (including tuberculosis) and fungi and sent for cytology.

SEVERE HYPERTENSION

A sudden increase in blood pressure or pressure consistently in the 200/120 range may produce severe headache. These headaches are occipital and often occur early in the morning. Patients become drowsy and have seizures and focal neurological signs in addition to papilledema when the blood pressure is sufficiently elevated.

HEADACHE OF ANEMIA

Anemia associated with hypoxemia of the brain may lead to dilated intracranial blood vessels and headache. John Graham stated that headaches were more likely to follow an acute drop in hemoglobin rather than a gradual one.

LYME DISEASE

Patients with acute Lyme disease may develop a recent-onset severe headache. Classic cases are easy to diagnosis. If a patient spends time in woods with a high population of deer, gets bitten by a tiny deer tick, and develops a bulls-eye rash with fever, malaise, and joint pains with or without weakness on one side of the face or a radiculopathy, the diagnosis is fairly certain. If a patient comes from such an area and has none of the above symptoms but has recent-onset headache, a titer for Lyme disease should be drawn. If Lyme disease is strongly suspected and the titer is negative, another titer should be drawn in 1 to 2 months or a lumbar puncture should be performed to check the CSF for *Borrelia burgdorferi* antibodies, or both. Most infectious disease experts do not administer treatment unless *Borrelia burgdorferi* infection is documented or strongly suspected. Acute infections are treated with doxycycline, and tertiary infections are treated with intravenous ceftriaxone (Rocephin) for 2 to 4 weeks.

Many patients who are accurately diagnosed and effectively treated and who no longer have active Lyme disease continue to have moderately severe, bilateral, steady head pains that lasts for months. These headaches can be effectively treated with intravenous, repetitive D.H.E. 45 followed by daily, small doses of antidepressants and vasoactive medication.

POST-SEIZURE HEADACHE

Seizure patients awaken from an epileptic attack with confusion and a generalized, moderately severe, throbbing headache that lasts for several hours and usually resolves spontaneously.

HEADACHE RELATED TO HYPOXIA

Patients who do not get enough oxygen, either because of lung disease or elevated carbon monoxide levels, usually develop a severe headache, which is possibly related to dilated cerebral vessels. Headaches also occur at high altitudes and are associated with acute mountain sickness. Altitudes greater than 7000 to 8000 feet above sea level are those more likely to be associated with symptoms of mountain sickness.

Mountain sickness occurs within a few hours of exposure to low oxygen tension and is probably related to dilated cerebral arteries in milder cases and to cerebral edema in more severe ones. When severe, mountain sickness may be associated with irritability, depression, insomnia, and even cerebral hemorrhage. Treatment includes moving to a lower altitude, breathing oxygen, and administration of acetazolamide (Diamox) 250 mg tid and/or dexamethasone (Decadron) 4 mg tid.

SEXUAL HEADACHE (ORGASMIC OR COITAL HEADACHE)

Sexual headache is a variety of exertional headache. It presents as a severe headache that occurs at the height of sexual arousal. The headache is usually bilateral, severe, and throbbing and varies in duration from minutes to hours. Patients who have this headache must be evaluated for subarachnoid hemorrhage and other serious illness the first time it occurs. If the headache recurs, it is usually benign in nature. If it is associated with vomiting, loss of consciousness, meningeal irritation, and residual pain on the following day, a subarachnoid hemorrhage is more likely than benign orgasmic cephalalgia. Etiology is variable, but the headache is usually the result of dilated blood vessels or strained muscles in the cervical and shoulder area.

POST-TRAUMATIC HEADACHE

Head injuries most frequently result from falls or motor vehicle accidents; alcohol often plays a significant role. Sports and industrial accidents account for the remainder of cases. The severity and duration of the headache are often unrelated or inversely related to the severity of the head injury. In addition to the headache, patients usually develop a post–head trauma syndrome, which is characterized by poor memory, reduced attention span, confusion, inability to think clearly, apathy, irritability and depression, insomnia, light-headedness, dizziness and vertigo, decreased libido, and other psychological problems.

Head pain and associated symptoms occur at the time of injury, but they often develop on the second day or several days later. In rare cases, symptoms may develop after several weeks or even months following the initial injury.

A typical closed-head injury is characterized by tearing or stretching of the nerve fibers because of shearing forces and by hemorrhage and edema. The headache is usually bilateral and constant but may be intermittent and can involve any part of the head. Patients usually describe it as a deep, pressing, squeezing ache; less frequently, the headache may be described as throbbing or pounding. Soon after a traumatic event, headache secondary to closed-head injury is associated with nausea; bending over, straining, and mild exercise may aggravate the headache. Some patients develop typical migraine, tension-type headache syndromes, or nonspecific headaches following head injury. Although less likely to occur, the onset of cluster headache occasionally follows head injury.

Although such studies are usually unrevealing, CT or MRI scans should be performed to rule out hemorrhage or edema

when a head injury appears severe enough to warrant it or if symptoms are ambiguous.

Antidepressants effectively relieve headache pain for most patients with headache secondary to closed-head injury. For patients whose headaches have a migraine component, preventive migraine drugs such as β-blockers, calcium channel blockers, and anticonvulsants such as Depakote should be tried. Biofeedback may help, as may other types of behavioral therapy.

Acute care medication often fails to provide pain relief, and patients must be counseled about limiting the use of pain medication. Midrin, Cafergot, D.H.E. 45, and Imitrex may provide pain relief, as may Fiorinal and Fioricet. Butorphanol nasal spray (Stadol NS) may relieve some patients' pain, but in most cases opiates should not be used on a daily basis.

Post-traumatic head pain decreases over several weeks, but complete relief of headache symptoms may take months or years. Ongoing legal action may appear to prolong the period of pain and disability.

Some patients develop a severe and chronic headache problem that does not respond to any therapeutic intervention; these patients may require expert care and even inpatient treatment.

HYPOGLYCEMIA AND HEADACHE

When diabetics become hypoglycemic because of an excess of insulin, they develop headache along with autonomic symptoms. Nondiabetics with relative hypoglycemia after eating a large, high-carbohydrate meal or after not eating for a long time usually get headache that is not accompanied by low blood glucose levels. The headache is usually bilateral and steady, and it may not improve for several hours after treatment. Missing or delaying a meal often triggers a headache in migraineurs. Migraineurs can avoid such headaches by eating at regular intervals and avoiding high-carbohydrate meals. Most physicians do not make a diagnosis of hypoglycemia, except when it is documented by a strictly defined and abnormally low serum glucose level on a 5-hour glucose tolerance test.

ENDOCRINE CAUSES OF HEADACHE

Any endocrine dysfunction or metabolic abnormality may result in headache. Patients with hypothyroidism, hyperparathyroidism, and hyperprolactinemia associated with pituitary adenoma all can develop mild, deep, steady, unrelenting headache. Occasionally, treatment of prolactinoma with bromocriptine (Parlodel) can produce headache.

GIANT CELL ARTERITIS (TEMPORAL ARTERITIS)

Patients with temporal arteritis often have headache, visual dysfunction, malaise, fever, and diffuse weakness. A typical patient is female and older than 55 years of age who presents with new onset of headache on one side of the head, most often over the temporal artery. The temporal artery pulse is decreased, and the artery feels firm and beaded and is tender to the touch.

Patients with giant cell arteritis have an elevated sedimentation rate and frequently have a history of claudication of the jaw. An abnormal temporal artery biopsy confirms the diagnosis. Note that the biopsy specimen requires meticulous attention on the part of a pathologist because there are often skip areas, so the entire specimen should be analyzed histopathologically. The treatment for temporal arteritis is 6 to 12 months of medium-dose oral steroids.

PAINFUL OPHTHALMOPLEGIA (TOLOSA-HUNT SYNDROME)

Patients with this condition present with a steady or throbbing pain behind one eye followed by decreased movement of the eye. This may persist for several weeks and often remits spontaneously. It is thought to be

caused by an inflammation in the cavernous sinus but could be caused by a structural lesion. The treatment is corticosteroid therapy.

SINUS HEADACHE

Although sinus headache occurs rarely compared with the number of people who think they have it, it can occur and the diagnosis can be missed. Most people who think they have chronic sinus headache actually have chronic tension-type headache, and they respond to sinus medication initially. Eventually, they develop analgesic rebound headache. Even when patients have a mild sinus problem, adequate treatment for the problem does not usually relieve the headache.

Acute sinusitis, however, often produces dramatic painful symptoms and must be treated quickly and may set off a migraine attack. Acute sinusitis is caused by an infection in one of the sinus cavities and may produce pain in various parts of the head or face, usually in a cheek, behind or over an eye, in the teeth, or on top of the head (Fig. 3–2). It is usually accompanied by fever, pain in the nose or sinus, a redness of the skin over the sinus, and yellow-green discharge from the nostrils and the back of the throat. Treatment consists of antibiotic therapy with sinus drainage.

Chronic sinusitis is a result of a low-grade inflammation in any one of the sinuses. Pain patterns are similar to those of acute sinus disease, but they are usually less severe and are not associated with an acute febrile illness. Patients complain of thickened secretions, aching over the sinuses, and postnasal drip. Diagnosis is at times difficult and may be missed by sinus x-rays. A CT scan of the sinuses or endoscopy should be performed to confirm the diagnosis.

When a patient has recent-onset, severe, bilateral headache that has not been diagnosed, sphenoid or ethmoid sinusitis should be considered and ruled out by a CT scan of the sinuses and consultation with an otolaryngologist.

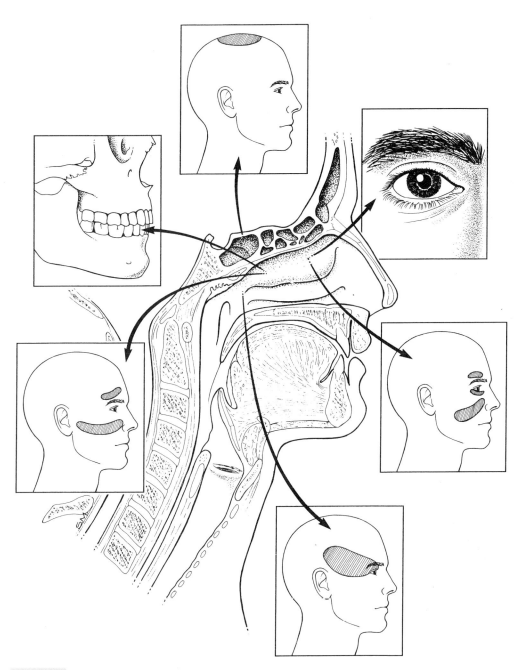

Figure 3-2

Radiation of sinus pain. Diagram of the areas of the skull, face, and teeth to which pain from different areas of the nose and sinuses can radiate.

EYE STRAIN HEADACHE

Some patients develop mild, bilateral headache when they use their eyes too intensely or fail to get glasses or change their prescription when necessary. Overlooking this potential cause of headache often results in unnecessary consultations and expensive, unrevealing testing before a diagnosis is made.

DENTAL DISEASE

Dental disease usually causes unilateral upper- or lower-jaw pain that may radiate into the cheek or eye. One or more teeth may be sensitive to cold or painful upon biting. Most dentists, endodontists, and oral surgeons make accurate diagnoses. In some cases, however, a tooth may be extracted or operated upon when the pain is neurological in origin.

TEMPOROMANDIBULAR JOINT DISEASE

Temporomandibular joint (TMJ) disorders are becoming a popular diagnosis. Almost everyone has a click or pop in the TMJ, and general dentists often consider this abnormal and a possible cause of headache. Over 80% of patients treated in a tertiary care headache clinic have been told by some previous physician they had TMJ syndrome; some have been treated for it but continue to experience headaches.

Disorders of the TMJ are usually related to acute muscle disorders (myofascial pain dysfunction), occlusal problems, joint inflammation, or structural defect. Pain usually occurs in and around a temporomandibular joint and may radiate from there to the temple, to the frontal area, or into the jaw. It is often worse on chewing, yawning, or grinding the teeth; clenching the teeth or opening the mouth widely may elicit pain.

Patients who present with symptoms that suggest TMJ dysfunction should be referred to a to a TMJ specialist. Some of the many forms of treatment are controversial, but we believe that biofeedback training and other behavioral techniques often help, and they are free of side effects.

Unless significant structural abnormality is present, TMJ disorders should be treated conservatively. Dental appliances, muscle relaxants, heat, antidepressants, and anti-inflammatory medications may be beneficial in many cases. Patients should avoid surgery unless more than one TMJ specialist suggests it.

ALLERGY AND HEADACHE

Food sensitivities in adults are usually the result of chemical reactions rather than true immunoglobulin E–mediated allergies. It has not been proven that true allergy causes migraine in adults. There have been some reports in children, however, that very strict elimination diets may be successful, suggesting an etiologic role for allergy. When patients have an acute allergic reaction to grasses, pollens, ragweed, or other seasonal allergens, their stuffed noses and sinuses can lead to an acute headache that may respond to antihistamines. Rarely, however, do patients with migraine benefit from allergy testing and treatment.

Some patients with allergic rhinitis complain of paranasal discomfort and headache. They often have symptoms such as rhinorrhea, sneezing, and nasal congestion. Vasomotor rhinitis caused by temperature changes, exercise, and change in barometric pressure may cause similar symptoms.

CHRONIC FATIGUE SYNDROME

Many patients develop chronic fatigue syndrome characterized by low-grade fever, myalgia, extreme fatigue, headache, and depression. They often have high serum titers of the Epstein-Barr virus that are usually chronically elevated.

This syndrome bears many similarities to fibromyalgia, which causes myalgia, arthralgia, and multiple tender points in muscles (trigger points). These patients typically have bilateral, steady, chronic, tension-type headache. Treatment with antidepressants may offer at least some relief. Muscle relaxants such as cyclobenzaprine (Flexeril) can be helpful, and education is essential, as the symptoms are often chronic and do not respond well to treatment. Before making the diagnosis, it is important to rule out organic disease such as Lyme disease, anorexia, and thyroid dysfunction.

TRIGEMINAL NEURALGIA (TIC DOULOUREUX)

Trigeminal neuralgia is characterized by severe, paroxysmal pain that is usually confined to one division of the trigeminal nerve on one side of the face. Often triggered by a touch to the face, speaking, eating, or brushing the teeth, patients describe it as an electric shock or intolerable paroxysm of pain that is severe and lancinating and usually persists for as long as 2 to 4 minutes. The pain may recur several times per day and is often worse in the morning. Symptoms may last for several weeks or months before disappearing for months at a time. Trigeminal neuralgia can become more chronic over time.

Although it usually affects only one division of the fifth cranial (trigeminal) nerve, it may occasionally affect two divisions. The second (maxillary) and third (mandibular) divisions are more commonly involved than the first (ophthalmic) division. Neurological examination and most tests such as MRI and brain stem auditory evoked response (BAER) are normal. This syndrome is caused occasionally by multiple sclerosis and can also be caused by pressure on the fifth nerve from a tumor or vascular lesion.

Medical treatment is often effective with the use of carbamazepine (Tegretol), phenytoin (Dilantin), baclofen (Lioresal), clonazopam (Klonopin), and antidepressants. Topical capsaicin (Zostrix), a hot pepper extract which depletes substance P, can be helpful.

When medical treatment is not successful, surgical intervention may be effective. The two most common types are percutaneous denervation of the gasserian (fifth) ganglion or suboccipital craniectomy with microvascular decompression. The latter procedure sometimes uncovers an arterial loop or vein pressing on a branch of the fifth nerve.

"ICE-CREAM" HEADACHE

The ice-cream headache is a headache that occurs in response to a cold stimulus and lasts for 10 to 30 seconds. It is characterized by very severe pain at the bridge of the nose, behind or beneath the eyes, or in the upper throat. It is triggered by a cold stimulus at the back of the throat, which probably stimulates the fifth or the ninth cranial nerve, or both. The headache occurs more frequently in migraine patients than in others and is a benign condition. It can be avoided by taking a small amount of ice cream and letting it dissolve in the mouth before swallowing; the pain may be also be brought on by cold liquids.

HEADACHE ASSOCIATED WITH FEVER

Any febrile illness, whether viral or due to serious septicemia, can cause severe headache. The headache is usually a deep, dull, generalized, throbbing pain, but may be worse in any part of the head, especially occipitally. It is almost always made worse by effort, bending, or coughing, and usually worsens as the day progresses.

Indications for Diagnostic Work-Up in Headache

A young, healthy patient with a clear-cut history suggestive of migraine may not need further work-up. However, patients who have migraine with aura, complicated migraine, chronic tension-type headache, slowly worsening headache syndromes, and unusual types of headache, especially those that are unilateral and associated with any neurologic symptomatology, should be investigated. A first attack of what appears to be migraine should probably be investigated. Patients with basilar artery migraine and other significant neurological history should have further work-up.

Patients with any of the red flags or changing headache as described earlier in this chapter should have a work-up. A CT or MRI scan should be performed to rule out structural disease when appropriate. If the headache is severe and of sudden onset, a CT scan should be performed immediately, followed by a spinal tap. CT scans are more accurate in detecting acute subarachnoid hemorrhage and focal bleeding than are MRI scans. When the CT scan is negative, a lumbar puncture may reveal subarachnoid bleeding or infection, even without suggestive clinical signs. Careful attention to opening and closing pressure is essential. Spinal fluid should be analyzed for cells, protein, glucose, and VDRL, antigens identified, and a culture begun. The spinal fluid should also be observed for color and clarity.

Intravenous contrast material to enhance CT scanning is usually helpful in uncovering tumors, AVMs, and other lesions. It is not required if hemorrhage is present on non-contrast scans. Contrast is not usually needed in MRI imaging except in special circumstances. MRI scans much more accurately detect Arnold-Chiari malformations, small lesions of the ventricular system, brain stem lesions, microadenomas of the pituitary gland, and unidentified bright objects, which are seen in migraineurs but may also represent demyelinating or tiny vascular lesions. MRI scans are preferable in evaluation of chronic headache conditions.

Sinus disease can usually be detected with sinus x-rays, but a CT scan of the sinuses provides more information. Lesions at the base of the skull and in the posterior fossa are best identified with thin cuts taken by MRI.

CRANIAL X-RAYS

Skull x-rays are rarely performed today; sinus x-rays may still be helpful. Plain x-rays of the cervical spine are helpful in diagnosing arthritis and fracture but not disc disease.

RADIONUCLIDE SCANS

Although radionuclide scans are helpful, they are rarely performed today because MRI provides a more detailed, accurate picture. Single photon emission computed tomography (SPECT) and positron emission tomography (PET) are still experimental in the evaluation of headache. SPECT findings may be abnormal in severe head trauma.

CEREBRAL ANGIOGRAPHY

Cerebral angiography is required only occasionally in the diagnosis of headache conditions. It should be considered when attempting to rule out vascular abnormalities such as aneurysms, cerebral arteritis, arteriovenous malformations, and carotid artery stenosis, occlusion, or dissection. Patients with migraine should not have direct carotid artery punctures for angiography. Intra-arterial injections of contrast media into any blood vessel that leads to a migraine patient's brain should be avoided, as it may cause arterial spasm and transient ischemic attack. MRA may provide adequate information without being invasive.

ELECTROENCEPHALOGRAPHY (EEG)

The use of electroencephalography in migraine is controversial. Many abnormalities have been described over the years, but not all neurologists find this test helpful or agree on interpretation of findings. Paroxysmal and sharp electroencephalograms in migraine patients may suggest the use of anticonvulsant medication. Epileptiform patterns are occasionally discovered, especially in children. Asymmetrical electroencephalograms may suggest the need for CT or MRI scanning to rule out focal lesions. It should be ordered if there is a history of seizures, loss of consciousness, head trauma, or sudden spells of dizziness, headache, or presyncope.

BLOOD TESTS

A complete blood count is helpful to diagnose anemia and other more serious hematological conditions, including reactions to medication. A general chemistry profile can detect hidden medical conditions such as hepatitis and renal dysfunction. Both of these tests should be done periodically when patients are on medications such as carbamazepine and divalproex sodium (Depakote). A measurement of the erythrocyte sedimentation rate helps to rule out temporal or giant cell arteritis and other inflammatory conditions. Titers for Lyme disease should be taken in areas where Lyme disease is common, even without obvious exposure, and a thyroid-stimulating hormone (TSH) test should be done to rule out thyroid disease. Other tests can be performed when indicated.

EVOKED POTENTIALS

Evoked potentials can be important diagnostic tests for certain neurological diseases; they are abnormal in migraine, suggesting excitability of the cortex. Flash visual evoked potentials may be abnormal in migraine. Brain stem auditory evoked responses can detect brain stem dysfunction, especially in multiple sclerosis, and can also be abnormal in migraine with and without aura, basilar artery migraine, and cluster headache.

TRANSCRANIAL DOPPLER

Transcranial Doppler evaluations have shown abnormal findings in cluster headache and migraine and are helpful in detecting intracranial vascular abnormalities.

THERMOGRAPHY

Some of the world's top headache researchers, including Lance and Anthony in Sydney, Australia; Kudrow in Los Angeles; Friedman (deceased) in New York; Mathew in Houston; and Swerdlow in Winter Park, Florida, have found significant abnormalities in thermography of the head and face in headache patients. Changes are detected interictally, and more significant abnormalities may be found during a migraine or cluster attack. Migraine patients have asymmetrical heat in the supraorbital areas and usually have cold noses and cheeks. Cluster patients usually have very warm noses and cheeks and a cold spot over the painful eye. Showing thermograms that provide graphic evidence of altered physiology helps patients to realize that their headaches are not "all in their minds."

In short, clinicians should become concerned and conduct appropriate examinations and testing when a primary headache pattern changes significantly; when a patient presents with first and/or worst headache; when a head injury may underlie headache pain; or when other medical problems or neurological dysfunctions are suspected.

SUGGESTED READINGS

Behrens MM: Headaches associated with disorders of the eye. *Med Clin North Am.* 1978;62:507.

Brisman R: Trigeminal neuralgia and other facial pains: Diagnosis, natural history, and nonsurgical treatment. In Brisman R (ed): *Neurosurgical and Medical Management of Pain: Trigeminal Neuralgia, Chronic Pain, and Cancer Pain.* Boston: Kluwer Academic. 1989; 25.

Day JW, Raskin NH: Thunderclap headache: Symptom of unruptured cerebral aneurysm. *Lancet.* 1986;2: 1247.

Edmeads J: Headaches in cerebrovascular disease. *Postgrad Med.* 1987;81(8):191.

Forsyth PA, Posner JB: Headaches in patients with brain tumors: A study of 111 patients. *Neurology.* 1993;43:1678.

Gfeller JD, Chibnall MS, Duckro PN: Postconcussion symptoms and cognitive functioning in posttraumatic headache patients. *Headache.* 1994;34:503.

Hatfield WB: Headache associated with metabolic and systemic disorders. *Med Clin North Am.* 1978; 62(3)451.

Marcelis J, Silberstein SD: Spontaneous low cerebral spinal fluid pressure headache. *Headache* 1990; 30:192.

Porter M, Jankovic J: Benign coital cephalalgia: Differential diagnosis and treatment. *Arch Neurol.* 1981;38:710.

Raskin NH: Lumbar puncture headache: A review. *Headache.* 1990;30(4):197.

Stammberger H, Wolf G: Headaches and sinus disease:

The endoscopic approach. *Ann Otol Rhinol Laryngol.* 1988(Suppl 134):3.

Solomon S, Guglielmo-Cappa K: The headache of temporal arteritis. *J Am Geriatr Soc.* 1987;35:163.

Tunkel AR, Wispelwey B, Scheld WM: Bacterial meningitis: Recent advances in pathophysiology and treatment. *Ann Intern Med.* 1990;112:610.

Verweij RD, Wijdicks EFM, van Gijn J: Warning headache in aneurysmal subarachnoid hemorrhage. *Arch Neurol.* 1988;45:1019.

Wijdicks EFM, Kerkhoff H, van Gijn J: Long-term follow-up with 71 patients with thunderclap headache mimicking subarachnoid hemorrhage. *Lancet.* 1988; 2:68.

CHAPTER FOUR

Pathophysiology of Headache

In the 17th century, Sir Thomas Willis ascribed headache to increased blood flow to the head that distended vessels and put pressure on the brain's nerve fibers. Although questioned at various times, Willis' *vascular* theory remained the leading hypothesis as to the cause of head pain until fairly recently.

In the 19th century, however, Liveing and Gowers believed that "nerve storms" resembling epilepsy were the cause, and that changes in blood vessels were secondary events. The vascular versus *neurogenic* theories of causality have been hotly debated since then.

In 1938, Graham (Fig. 4–1) and Wolff, two of the best known headache researchers in the first half of the 20th century, published a paper entitled *Mechanism of Migraine Headache: An Action of Ergotamine Tartrate.* They believed that the aura warning of migraine was caused by constriction of intracerebral arteries that decreased blood flow to the visual cortex in the occipital lobe, and that the pain which followed was the result of distention of the external carotid system with compression of nerves in the carotid artery wall. They demonstrated that ergotamine tartrate both decreased the pulse amplitude in the superficial temporal

artery, which is an end branch of the external carotid artery system, and decreased head pain.

In his now-classic text entitled *Headache and Other Head Pain*, published in 1963, Wolff suggested that these vascular changes might be secondary to a central process. He also suggested that the central process had at least two necessary components to produce headache: the release of edema-producing chemicals from nerve fibers, and vasodilation.

The exact cause of head pain is still controversial. Many researchers believe that an intracerebral, meningeal, or extracranial vascular component is associated with release of humoral agents that mediate biochemical changes. Others maintain that all clinical aspects of migraine, including the head pain, are the result of central processes that occur in the brain and brain stem.

Any encompassing theory to explain the pathophysiology of migraine must account for such widely divorced symptoms as the premonitory ones that include mood changes, increased appetite, and yawning; occasional focal neurologic signs and symptoms (such as hemiparesis, hemisensory syndrome) or visual aura (such as fortification spectra, scotomata, or photopsias [flashes of light]);

37

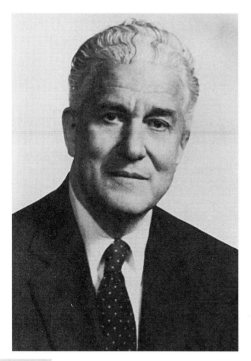

Figure 4–1

Dr. John Graham was one of the grandfathers of headache treatment and research in America. He was the director of the John Graham Headache Center in Boston and along with Harold Wolff did several pivotal clinical studies on headache patients. He was a great teacher, mentor, and researcher, a selfless healer, and a special human being. He was born in 1919 and died in 1990.

and pain in the head, often in or behind the eye, and in some cases involving the face or neck.

A discussion of the scientific evidence contributing to pathophysiological mechanisms follows, along with a summary of the three major theories that explain them: the vascular and central hypotheses, and the theory of dysfunction of the trigeminovascular system.

The Origin of Head Pain

Studies conducted by Ray and Wolff in 1940 established which areas inside and outside the cranium were responsible for head pain. Brain substance is insensitive to pain; however, the meninges, the proximal intracerebral arteries, the veins and venous sinuses, and the external carotid system are all pain-sensitive, as are cranial nerves 5, 7, 9, and 10. It has also been shown that struc-

tures in the posterior fossa, the upper cervical roots and their peripheral nerves, and muscles in the back of the head and neck usually refer pain to the back of the head. On the other hand, the upper cervical roots and the greater occipital nerve sometimes refer pain to the frontal area and the ipsilateral eye.

CEREBRAL BLOOD FLOW AND CORTICAL SPREADING DEPRESSION

Since 1981, many studies have examined the degree to which changes in cerebral blood flow and in electrical activity precede or trigger a migraine attack.

Working in Copenhagen, Denmark, Olesen and associates (1981) studied patients with migraine with aura. Their research demonstrated that migraineurs have a decrease in cerebral blood flow that begins in the occipital region and extends slowly anteriorly as a wave of "spreading oligemia," traveling across the cortex at 2 to 3 mm per minute (Fig. 4–2). This phenomenon does not follow vascular boundaries, lasts for several hours, and is followed by hyperemia. The aura begins while the cerebral blood flow is diminished; the headache also begins during this phase.

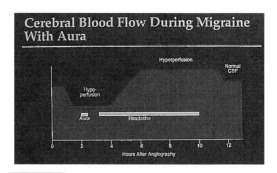

Figure 4–2

Changes in cerebral blood flow during a migrainous aura and headache attack based on studies by Professor Jes Olesen from Copenhagen. According to many scientific studies performed on migraine patients by Professor Olesen, cerebral blood flow decreases prior to the aura and remains decreased during the entire aura and the early phase of the headache. It then increases during the later headache phase. Dr. Olesen describes an oligemia in the posterior cerebral cortex prior to migraine pain; however, he feels there is no direct relationship between blood flow changes and headache. (From Olesen J: Cerebral and extracranial circulatory disturbances in migraine: Pathophysiological implications. *Cerebrovasc Brain Metab Rev.* 1991;31:1–28; Courtesy of Sandoz Pharmaceuticals Corp.)

Olesen did not believe that there was true cerebral hypoxia. Skyhøj-Olsen and colleagues (1987), on the other hand, maintained that changes in cerebral blood flow described by Olesen were artifactual. No such changes in blood flow have ever been reported in migraine without aura (previously called common migraine).

Cortical spreading depression was first described by Leão in 1944 while he conducted research at Harvard. He theorized that a slowly spreading wave of electrical depression that follows a sudden increase in electrical activity in the posterior part of the brain in rabbits was analogous to an electrical event in migraineurs. Welch and coworkers (1987 and 1990) used magnetoencephalography to measure electrical potentials and magnetic waves emanating from the brains of patients experiencing migraine and found that they had transient decreases in electrical cortical potentials which appear to be the human correlate of the spreading depression proposed by Leão. Welch also found low levels of intracellular magnesium at the beginning of a migraine attack, a tantalizing hint that there may be a discernible factor that results in electrical irritability of the cortex. The exact relationship of these findings to the beginning of a migraine attack is not yet clear.

Woods and associates (1995) described a patient with migraine who had bilateral hypoperfusion, seen on positron emission tomography (PET) scan, that spread anteriorly from the occipital lobes, possibly as the result of spreading depression.

BIOCHEMICAL CHANGES ASSOCIATED WITH MIGRAINE

Migraine patients' platelets are characterized by hyperaggregability. Much of the body's serotonin is in the platelets. During a migraine attack, platelet serotonin increases prior to onset of headache and decreases during the headache phase. This leads to increased excretion of 5-hydroxyindoleacetic acid (5-HIAA), the main metabolite of serotonin, in the urine following a migraine attack. Gawel and coworkers (1979) found

evidence of a platelet release reaction in migraine accompanied by an increase in β-thromboglobulin during the headache phase, suggesting platelet activation.

Serotonin (5-Hydroxytryptamine [5-HT])

Anthony and colleagues (1967) were the first to report a serotonin-releasing factor in the blood during a migraine attack. After serotonin is released from platelets, it has a potent vasoconstrictor effect. Rather than acting alone, serotonin may be one of a number of chemicals, such as neuropeptides, that work in concert to sensitize blood vessel walls to painful dilation.

At least seven 5-HT receptors have been identified. These receptors fall into four main groups and are found in the meninges, in certain layers of the cortex, in deeper structures in the brain, and, most commonly, in brain stem nuclei. There are two important serotonin receptors in headache: one may terminate an acute attack; the other may prevent one. When stimulated, the 5-HT$_1$ receptors can terminate an acute migraine attack; 5-HT$_2$ receptors can prevent migraine attacks from occurring when they are blocked (antagonized) on a daily basis, making them useful as migraine-preventive agents.

This information helps explain why both serotonin agonists *and* antagonists are useful in treating migraine. Specifically, such medications as sumatriptan (Imitrex), dihydroergotamine (D.H.E. 45), and ergotamine tartrate (Cafergot) that **stimulate** 5-HT$_1$ receptors are useful in treating acute attacks. Others, such as cyproheptadine (Periactin), methysergide (Sansert), several tricyclic antidepressants, and some calcium channel blockers **antagonize** or downregulate 5-HT$_2$ receptors and often help prevent migraine. These medications will be discussed in greater depth in Chapter 6.

Serotonin receptors are important in understanding the trigeminovascular system and its relationship to migraine, as will be explained.

Many other neurotransmitters and neuro-

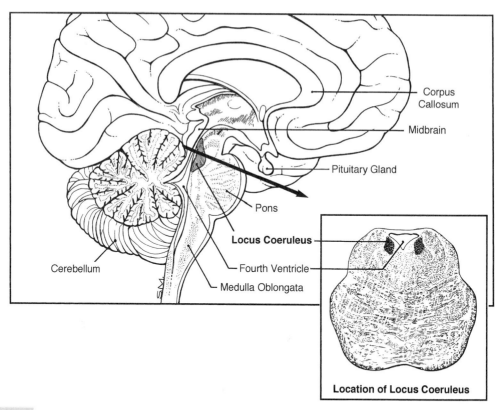

Figure 4–3

Representation of the locus coeruleus located in the dorsal pons just below and lateral to the floor of the fourth ventricle. This bilateral structure releases noradrenaline.

chemicals are involved in the migraine process. Catecholamines such as noradrenaline (also called norepinephrine) may be important. Noradrenaline is found in the locus coeruleus (Fig. 4–3), in the pons of the brain stem. It mediates both vasoconstriction and vasodilation in addition to playing a role in the release of free fatty acids, a process that signals platelets to release serotonin.

Dopamine, another catecholamine, may play a role in headache. Dopamine receptor antagonists, such as metoclopramide (Reglan), may diminish headache and are often used to treat nausea and vomiting. Excitatory amino acids, such as glutamate, may set up an electrical reaction in the cortex that could induce spreading depression and lead to headache. Multiple vasoactive neuropeptides have been studied and are released at nerve terminals after electrical stimulation. Some of these agents are vasoconstrictors such as neuropeptide Y, and others are vasodilators such as calcitonin gene–related peptide (CGRP) and vasoactive intestinal polypeptide (VIP).

Certain specific insults to animals produce a marked increase in these polypeptides in the external jugular vein. The exact function of these peptides in the vascular events of migraine headache is unclear; however, histamine increases after a migraine headache and **may** be involved as a vasodilator in the migraine process. Even nitric oxide has been implicated with respect to its role as the endothelial releasing factor, which can contribute to vasodilation.

Many foods, such as ripened cheeses, red wine, liver, and yogurt, which contain *tyramine* (derived from tyrosine), may trigger a migraine headache in susceptible individuals, as may *chocolate,* which contains *phenylethylamine* (the amino acid derived from phenylalanine).

Endogenous *opioids* are believed to be among the chemical factors that regulate pain in migraineurs. Levels of β-endorphins, enkephalins, and dynorphins have been studied during and between migraine episodes. Findings have been conflicting and inconclusive. Sicuteri and colleagues (1983) reported that an injection of opioid-inhibiting naloxone shortened the duration of or stopped migraine aura in most patients.

Long-chain fatty acids derived from arachidonic acid, the prostaglandin, appear to be responsible for the pain, inflammation, and vasodilation of menstrually related migraine. Because nonsteroidal anti-inflammatory agents are prostaglandin inhibitors, such agents are frequently used in treatment of migraine headache attacks, especially around the time of menses.

Free fatty acids rise in fasting patients and are believed to cause headache in susceptible individuals. These agents may signal blood platelets to release serotonin.

The Central Theory

The central theory of the pathophysiology of migraine is based on several clinical and experimental factors. Migrainous aura, whether induced by 5-HT$_1$ receptors because of changes in blood flow or electrical cortical changes, is mediated by the visual cortex of the occipital lobes. We know that migraine may be associated with changes in cerebral blood flow and with changes in electrical cortical activity. These changes are evident in the increased amplitude of contingent negative variation and in the increased amplitude of visual evoked potentials in migraine patients.

The premonitory (prodromal) symptoms that may occur several hours or even as long as a day prior to the headache (such as mood changes, food craving, drowsiness, thirst, and yawning) suggest disruption in *hypothalamic* function (Fig. 4–4).

The autonomic nervous system is clearly involved in migraine and other types of headache. Pupillary changes are prominent in migraine; studies suggest that this is the result of a sympathetic dysfunction. Cluster headache is also characterized by major autonomic dysfunction.

Certain brain stem structures figure prom-

inently in the migraine story. The *locus coeruleus* is lateral to the floor of the fourth ventricle in the upper pons and holds numerous noradrenaline-containing neurons (see Fig. 4–3). Ascending projections from this nucleus to the cortex are related to the state of arousal and awareness. Descending projections are related to mechanisms of pain control. Stimulating the locus coeruleus decreases ipsilateral cerebral blood flow and increases blood flow in the external carotid artery system because of vasodilation. This process is mediated through the greater superficial petrosal branch of the facial (seventh) cranial nerve; these changes occur on the ipsilateral side to the stimulation and resemble the changes in migraine.

The *dorsal raphe nucleus* near the center of the midbrain (Fig. 4–5) contains a major collection of serotonin-containing neurons. It is characterized by diffuse interconnections projecting to the cortex, the hypothalamus, the lower brain stem, and to multiple blood vessels. According to Goadsby and colleagues (1991), stimulation of this nucleus increases cerebral blood flow by dilating both the internal and the external carotid circulations. Ascending projections from the midbrain raphe nucleus are also involved in sleep and neuroendocrine regulation.

Moskowitz (1990) has shown that stimulation of the trigeminal (fifth cranial) nerve dilates extracranial blood vessels possibly via release of vasoactive neuropeptides, such as substance P.

PAIN PATHWAYS

Pain from the periphery is transmitted along small myelinated and unmyelinated fibers that terminate in the dorsal horn of the spinal cord. There they synapse with secondary neurons that cross to the opposite side and ascend to the thalamus via the spinothalamic pathways. Fields (1987) has established that these pain signals are modulated in the dorsal horn by interneurons that contain enkephalin and γ-aminobutyric acid (GABA) (Fig. 4–6). These inhibitory interneurons are in turn influenced by de-

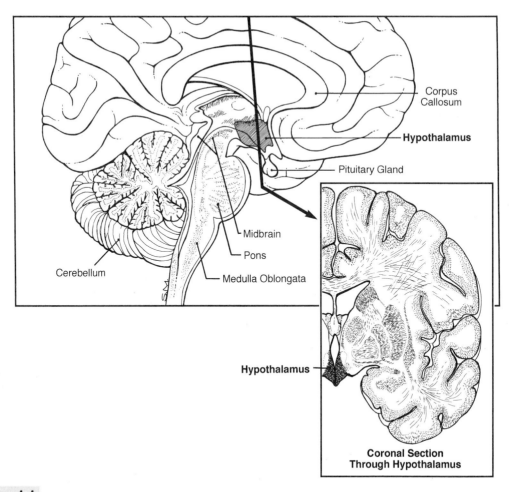

Figure 4–4

Representation of the hypothalamus, located at the base of the brain below the thalamus. Neural activity in the hypothalamus is thought to be responsible for the premonitory (prodromal) symptoms prior to a migraine attack. The biological clock is housed in the suprachiasmatic nucleus in the hypothalamus.

scending monoaminergic pathways: the serotonergic pathway emanating from the periaqueductal gray matter of the midbrain as well as the raphe nuclei, and the noradrenergic tract that originates in the locus coeruleus in the upper pons (Fig. 4–7).

According to Sicuteri, a deficiency of this monoaminergic descending influence could open the pain control gates and produce head and neck pain. Both the locus coeruleus and the raphe nuclei also have ascending pain-modulating pathways. These pathways influence the quality and emotional content of pain signals that project to the thalamus and the cortex. Sensory input from the head reaches the brain stem through the fifth, seventh, ninth, and tenth cranial nerves and the occipital nerves.

Fields has also described *on cells* and *off cells* in the medulla, which turn pain on and off. Most head pain is mediated by the trigeminal nerve in the pons, as will be described, but interconnections among the upper cervical nerves at their entry into the cervical spinal cord at C2 and C3 are significant and cannot be ignored.

Neurogenic Inflammation Theory

Moskowitz has shown that the trigeminovascular system is a key structure in the modulation of headache pain (Fig. 4–8). The *trigeminovascular system* arises in the meninges at the interface of the ends of the primary afferent small caliber C fibers of the

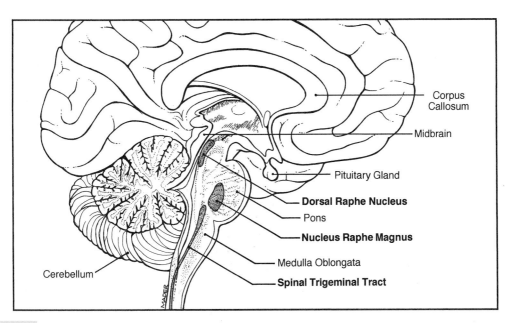

Figure 4–5

The dorsal raphe nucleus of the midbrain and the nucleus raphe magnus of the pons are two of the main serotonin-containing nuclei in the brain stem thought to be integrally involved in headache modulation.

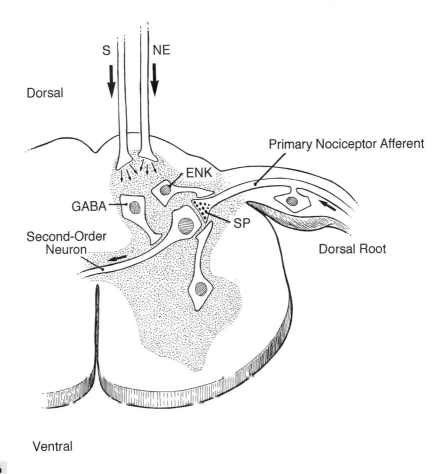

Figure 4–6

Modulation of different pain signals in the dorsal horn of the spinal cord by interneurons containing enkephalin (ENK) and γ-aminobutyric acid (GABA). NE, noradrenaline; S, serotonin; SP, substance P.

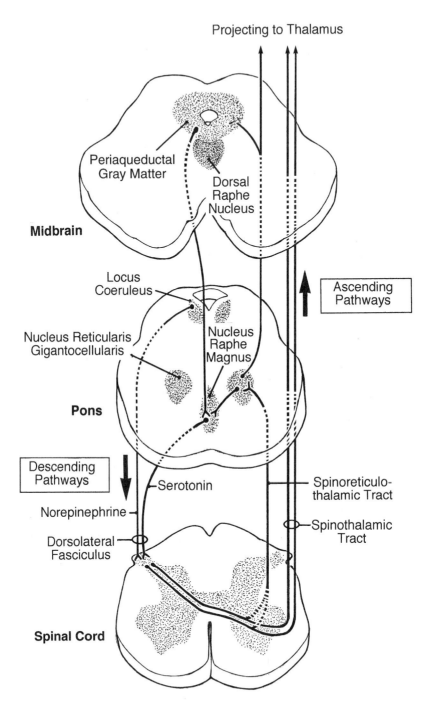

Figure 4–7

Representation of the descending serotonergic and noradrenergic modulatory pain pathways and the ascending pain pathways carrying impulses from the spinal cord to the thalamus.

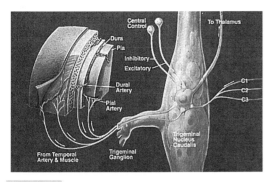

Figure 4–8

Representation of the trigeminovascular system consisting of the proximal central connections in the pons and the distal peripheral connections in the meninges of the trigeminal (fifth) cranial nerve. (After Olesen J: Clinical and pathophysiological observations in migraine and tension-type headache explained by integration of vascular, supraspinal, and myofascial inputs. *Pain.* 1991;46:125–132; Courtesy of Sandoz Pharmaceuticals Corp.)

fifth nerve whose cell bodies reside in the trigeminal ganglion and the adjacent dural blood vessels. Impulses travel along the fifth nerve to the ganglion outside the brain stem, into the pons, and descend and synapse in the trigeminal nucleus caudalis.

Ascending impulses reach the thalamus and then the cortex, where pain is registered. Moskowitz postulates that migraine-pain–producing neurogenic inflammation occurs at the interface of the end of the trigeminal nerve fibers and the dural arteries. This inflammation is caused by a release of neurotransmitters such as substance P, calcitonin gene–related peptide, and neurokinin A from the ends of the fifth nerve (Fig. 4–9). These neurotransmitters signal the adjacent dural blood vessels to dilate, extravasate plasma, and undergo vascular endothelial activation (Fig. 4–10). The resulting neurogenic inflammation sensitizes neurons and induces pain.

Electrical activity during the aura phase or at the beginning of the migraine attack is believed to depolarize the trigeminal nerve fibers adjacent to pial arteries and initiate the headache phase of the migraine attack. It has been demonstrated in guinea pigs that sumatriptan and dihydroergotamine block the release of substance P, caused by intravenous stimulation with capsaicin (extract of hot peppers) or electrical stimulation of C fibers, and prevent the formation of neuro-

genic inflammation and pain. This suggests that prejunctional stimulation of 5-HT$_1$ inhibitory fibers prevents the release of certain neuropeptides and blocks neurogenic inflammation.

Unification Theory

Lance and associates (1982, 1989) have proposed a unification theory of the pathogenesis of migraine that involves both the central nervous system and the peripheral blood vessels. Some process—possibly in the orbitofrontal and limbic cortices—triggers reactions in the brain stem noradrenergic system through the locus coeruleus and the serotonergic system through the dorsal raphe nucleus and the trigeminovascular system. This in turn alters the size of blood vessels, which may also trigger the trigeminal nerve impulses, leading to a vicious circle that intensifies the pain. Nausea and vomiting are probably caused by either dopamine or serotonin acting on the area postrema in the floor of the fourth ventricle in the medulla. Lance postulates that a segmental defect exists in the endogenous pain control pathways in migraine patients and cites as evidence spontaneous jabs of pain (ice-pick pains) and ice-cream headache (severe, short-lived vascular pain following the ingestion of cold food and drink) in mi-

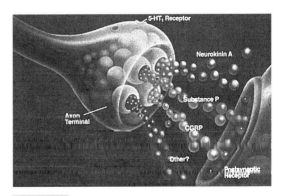

Figure 4–9

Representation of the release of neuropeptides such as substance P, calcitonin gene–related peptide (CGRP), and neurokinin A from presynaptic vesicles. Note the presynaptic serotonin (5-HT$_1$) receptor, which when stimulated prevents the release of these neuropeptides, thereby preventing the development of neurogenic inflammation. (Courtesy of Sandoz Pharmaceuticals Corp.)

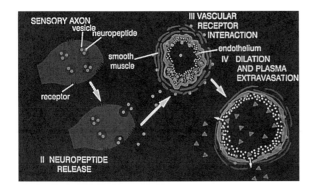

Figure 4-10

Representation of the end of the trigeminal nerve with its presynaptic vesicles and adjacent dural artery. When the presynaptic vesicles release their neurotransmitter contents, the adjacent vessel dilates, undergoes vascular endothelial activation, and extravasates plasma. This process is known as *neurogenic inflammation*. Stimulation of the distal primary afferent nerve produces pain signals, which reach the thalamus and induce pain. (Courtesy of Steven D. Silberstein, MD. Based on research by M. A. Moskowitz.)

graineurs in the area usually affected by headache.

Projections from the locus coeruleus to the cerebral cortex could produce cortical oligemia and possibly even spreading depression, resulting in the aura. This comprehensive theory explains many parts of the migraine process and also provides a rationale for the use of certain medications that block specific aspects of migraine's clinical progression.

MIGRAINE TRIGGERS

Vulnerability to developing a migraine headache is in part a function of inherited biological defects in the central nervous system. A variety of factors may trigger a migraine attack: it may be set off by numerous external and internal stimuli acting on a lowered biological threshold produced by some biochemical or physiological change. We have often used a stick-of-dynamite cartoon to explain the origin and trigger factors in migraine (Fig. 4–11). The stick of dynamite represents the inherited physiological dysfunction in the migraineur that produces biological vulnerability. In a vulnerable patient, a variety of triggering influences (detonators) can set off the explosion.

Hormonal Triggers

Hormonal fluctuation is a trigger factor in approximately 60% of women with migraine. Fourteen percent of women with migraine have their migraine attacks only during the menstrual cycle (true menstrual migraine). Both estrogen and progesterone levels begin to rise at the beginning of the menstrual cycle during menstrual flow (Fig. 4–12). Both levels increase at ovulation and remain high in the second half of the cycle (luteal phase); both decrease at the end of the cycle prior to the next period. Headaches appear to be triggered by falling levels of plasma estradiol-17β just prior to menses. Premenstrually, these headaches may be associated with mood changes, back pain, and breast tenderness and are part of the premenstrual syndrome (officially termed *late luteal phase dysphoric disorder*).

The headache that occurs in the perimenstrual period usually begins on the first day of menstruation but may occur up to 2 days before or 2 days after the start of menstruation. The exact mechanism is still unclear but seems to be related to falling estrogen levels and their effect on neurohormones, central mechanisms, hyperactive receptors, and blood vessels.

Studies by Somerville (1972) have shown that giving estrogen premenstrually delays the onset of migraine but does not affect menstruation; administration of progesterone delays the onset of menstruation but does not prevent a migraine attack. He concluded that estrogen withdrawal may trigger migraine in susceptible women. He found that oral administration of estrogen to women during the premenstrual portion of the cycle did not prevent menstrual migraine. However, several researchers have found that giving estradiol premenstrually via the Estraderm patch or sublingual Estrace may decrease or prevent attacks of menstrual migraine.

Migraine Trigger Factors

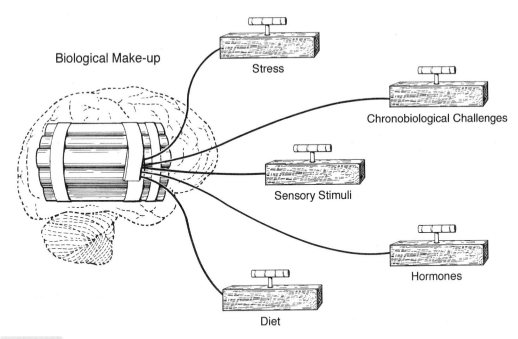

Figure 4–11

Representation of the various migraine trigger factors that can set off a headache in patients who have inherited the physiological susceptibility to migraine.

The high and relatively constant estrogen levels associated with pregnancy completely reverse the triggering aspect of falling estradiol levels that occur prior to menses. Plasma estradiol levels may be elevated 100-fold in late pregnancy. Many women have a flurry of headaches in the first trimester of pregnancy, usually followed by a marked decrease in migraine attacks in the final two. During the week following delivery, over 40% of migraineurs who had migraine before their pregnancy have a severe migraine attack, which may be caused by plummeting estradiol levels.

It is generally believed that women who take oral contraceptives are likely to experience increased frequency of migraine attacks. With some of the newer low-estrogen products, this phenomenon may be less of a problem. However, the cyclical dosing of estrogen appears to enhance normally fluctuating estrogen levels and to produce migraine.

Women whose headaches worsen when

Figure 4–12

Graph of the rise of estrogen following the beginning of a period and its fall prior to the next period. There is a rise of progesterone after ovulation and a fall prior to the next period. (From Rapoport A, Sheftell F: *Conquering Headache.* Hamilton, Ontario: Empowering Press. 1995.)

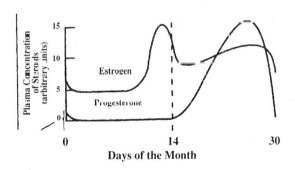

they take oral contraceptives usually improve over a period of 3 to 6 months when they discontinue oral contraceptives. We have seen isolated cases of severe headaches that began just 1 month after starting oral contraceptives; these patients' headaches did not improve for many months after discontinuation.

Menopause

There is no way to predict accurately whether and how a woman's headache pattern may change during and after menopause. In general, women seem to have an increase in frequency and severity of headaches in the years leading up to cessation of menstruation; some, but not all, note improvement after the menopause. This is greatly influenced by whether estrogen or progesterone (or both) is administered. From a headache standpoint alone, we have found the best situation is for patients to forego hormone replacement therapy (HRT). If HRT has been recommended by a woman's physician, then the lowest dose of estrogen possible, given on a daily and noncyclical constant basis, gives the best results.

The Estraderm patch seems to be better than oral estrogen, but pure estradiol in the form of Estrace 0.5 to 2 mg daily seems to work well. Most gynecologists feel that progesterone is necessary if the uterus is intact. If this is the case, we find that 2.5 mg of progesterone on a daily basis is far superior to 5 to 10 mg, 10 days per month, which is the usual way it is prescribed.

Food Triggers

Migraineurs are not usually allergic to foods (as mentioned in Chapter 3), but they sometimes react to chemicals in certain foods. We suggest that migraineurs be aware of foods that may set off migraine in susceptible individuals and that they try to limit those foods in their diet, especially during menses and ovulation (Table 4–1).

Alcohol is the most common food trigger. Any type of alcohol can trigger a migraine

Table 4–1
DIETARY FOOD TRIGGERS IN MIGRAINEURS

Food	Comments
Chocolate	
Canned eggs	
Nuts	
Peanut butter	
Onions	
Pizza	Avoid if possible
Sour cream	
Yogurt	
Herring	
Chicken livers	
Avocado	
NutraSweet (Equal)	
Ripened cheeses (eg, Cheddar, Gruyere, Brie, Camembert)	American, cottage, cream, and Velveeta (processed) cheeses are permissible
Vinegar	White vinegar is permissible
Anything fermented, pickled, or marinated	
Hot fresh breads, raised coffee cakes and donuts	Due to active yeast
Pods of broad beans (eg, lima, navy, pea)	
Monosodium glutamate	Any foods containing large amounts, eg, Chinese food
Citrus fruit	No more than one orange per day, for example
Bananas	No more than ½ banana per day
Pork	Limit intake
Tea, coffee, cola beverages	Avoid excessive amounts
Cured meats (eg, bologna, salami, pepperoni, summer sausage, hot dogs, bacon)	
Alcoholic beverages	**Avoid** if possible. Of all possible food triggers for migraine, alcohol is most frequently cited

Modified from *Helpful Hints for Headache Control.* The New England Center for Headache, Stamford, CT.

headache, probably by vasodilation, but wine, particularly red wine, and beer tend to be the worst offenders. Studies have shown that the darker colored alcohols (eg, scotch, bourbon, dark rum, and red wine) tend to cause more headaches than the lighter colored ones (eg, gin, vodka, light rum, and white wine).

Foods containing *tyramine*, which is produced from the amino acid tyrosine, such as aged cheeses, any type of food that is pickled or fermented, liver and paté, freshly baked breads, red wine, yogurt, figs, and bananas, are often migraine triggers.

Monosodium glutamate (MSG) is a frequent trigger for migraine and is also the cause of the *Chinese Restaurant Syndrome*, a headache associated with anxiety, dizziness, paresthesia of the neck and arms, and abdominal and chest pain. Foods that contain MSG include canned meats and soups, cookies, prepared diet foods, prepared frozen foods such as TV dinners, prepared gravies and gravy mixes, potato chips, salad dressings, and spices; MSG may be added to a wide variety of foods as a flavor enhancer. Food labels may be confusing; those that list hydrolized fat or hydrolized protein are suspect.

Chocolate sometimes triggers migraines because it contains *phenylethylamine,* a derivative of the amino acid phenylalanine. Women often crave chocolate during their menses, stacking one trigger upon another.

Nitrates, which preserve processed meats and prevent color deterioration, are found in bologna, salami, pepperoni, bacon, ham, hot dogs, presliced packaged meats, and many other processed meats. Nitrates dilate blood vessels and cause headache in susceptible individuals through the effects of nitric oxide. The *hot dog headache* is caused by the vasodilatory effects of nitrate-containing substances in a typical hot dog.

At the beginning of this century, the *gun powder headache* commonly afflicted workers in ammunition plants where gun powder containing *nitroglycerin* was used. Cardiac patients using sublingual nitroglycerin and other vasodilators frequently have headaches, as do hypertensive patients who take sublingual nifedipine (Procardia).

Aspartame is the major ingredient in NutraSweet (Equal) and often causes headaches in susceptible individuals. Aspartame is a synthetic chemical composed of two amino acids, aspartic acid and phenylalanine, plus methanol (wood alcohol, a poisonous substance that cannot be detoxified by the body). It is consumed by more than 100 million people in the United States, and it is 200 times sweeter than table sugar or sucrose.

Whereas caffeine may help to abort a migraine attack and is often found in off-the-shelf combination medications and in prescription headache medications, it can also increase headache via two mechanisms.

First, ingestion of too much caffeine seems to increase headache frequency. Too much is usually over 350 mg of caffeine per day, but there are some individuals who are susceptible to regular ingestion of even relatively small amounts (eg, 100 mg). The amount varies from person to person and probably is related to the sensitivity of the nervous system. Second, other patients have no trouble with a steady diet of 500 to 1000 mg of caffeine but get into trouble when they do not have their regular dose on time. This is a common cause of weekend headaches which occur on a Saturday or Sunday when many people take less caffeine. The headache occurs because people may switch to decaffeinated coffee on the weekend or get up later than usual and delay caffeine intake. This causes a caffeine withdrawal headache that is probably due to rebound vasodilation.

Caffeinism occurs at approximately 500 mg daily intake or more and includes sleeping difficulties, anxiety, irritability, palpitations, and nervousness (Table 4–2).

Environmental Triggers

Change in a migraineur's internal or external environment frequently produces an acute attack. Examples of internal change include hormonal fluctuation related to the menstrual cycle and alteration of circadian rhythms (eg, sleep-wake cycle). Examples of external change include the weather, seasons, changing time zones during air travel, altitude, and delaying or skipping meals.

Many migraineurs complain of *weather*-related headaches, but there is no scientific proof as to which factors may be responsible for this. Most patients say they get a headache when it is about to rain or is actually raining, when the barometric pressure is falling, or during other changes in weather patterns. Other patients have problems with high winds associated with positively changed small ionized particles in the air, extreme heat or cold, humidity, and other factors. Although patients differ among themselves in terms of weather triggers,

Table 4–2

CAFFEINE CONTENT OF BEVERAGES, FOODS, AND MEDICATIONS

Product	Example	Caffeine Content, mg
Cocoa and chocolate	Baking chocolate (1 oz)	35
	Chocolate candy bar	25
	Cocoa beverage (6 oz mixture)	10
	Milk chocolate (1 oz)	6
Coffee	Decaffeinated (5 oz)	2
	Drip (5 oz)	146
	Instant, regular (5 oz)	53
	Percolated (5 oz)	110
Off-the-shelf drugs	Anacin	32
	Extra-Strength Excedrin	65
	No-Doz tablets	100–200
	Vanquish	33
	Vivarin tablets	200
Prescription drugs	Darvon Compound-65	32.4
	Esgic	40
	Fioricet	40
	Fiorinal	40
	Norgesic	30
	Norgesic Forte	60
	Synalgos-DC	30
Soft drinks (12 oz)	7-Up/Diet 7-Up	0
	Coca-Cola	34
	Diet Pepsi	34
	Dr. Pepper	38
	Fresca	0
	Ginger Ale	0
	Hires Root Beer	0
	Mountain Dew	52
	Pepsi-Cola	37
	Tab	44
Tea	1-minute brew (5 oz)	9–33
	3-minute brew (5 oz)	22–46
	5-minute brew (5 oz)	20–50
	Canned ice tea (12 oz)	22–36

From Rapoport A, Sheftell F: *Conquering Headache.* Hamilton, Ontario: Empowering Press. 1995.

each individual always seems sensitive to the same triggers.

Sensory stimuli can trigger migraines. Patients report headaches set off by flickering lights; bright or flashing light; exposure to bright sunlight; or odors such as perfume, cleaning and other chemicals, and cigarette smoke. Extreme temperatures or loud noises are also triggers.

Other Triggers

Several *medications,* such as nitroglycerin, excessive tetracycline, large doses of vitamin-A, and specific serotonin re-uptake inhibitors such as fluoxetine (Prozac), can trigger migraines in some patients. Certain blood pressure medications such as nifedipine (Procardia) may have the same unwanted effect. It is important for the clinician to take a very careful history of medications taken, since these are easy to overlook in evaluating headache patients.

Stress has frequently and sometimes incorrectly been cited as a migraine trigger. Migraineurs and non-migraineurs alike may get tension-type headaches from increased stress. Although migraineurs sometimes have a worse headache during stressful periods, they usually do well during these periods and events and develop their headache when the stress lets up. Thus, migraineurs frequently complain of headaches in the evening after work, on weekends, at the beginning of vacations, and during let-down periods.

Other trigger factors are high altitude (over 8000 feet above sea level), physical exertion, sexual activity, head trauma, oral contraceptive intake, the perimenopausal years, menopause, and oversleeping or marked change in the chronobiological rhythms induced by an alteration of the sleep-wake cycle.

Finally, a confluence of trigger factors increases the potential for headaches in susceptible individuals. Such a situation may occur during air travel to different time zones, especially during holiday seasons. The multiple factors that trigger headaches may occur together and include plane travel, a change in chronobiological state during air travel to different time zones, and the excitement and changes in diet and sleep patterns that are associated with holiday periods.

The Pathophysiology of Tension-Type Headache

Tension-type headache was originally called tension headache because it was believed to be caused by tension of the muscles of the head, face, jaw, and neck. Most patients misunderstood this term and assumed that psychological tension was responsible for the headache; this misconception resulted in the popular myth that headache is caused by anxiety, nervousness, or depression. The International Headache Society (IHS) Classification separates tension-type headache into two categories: (1) those associated with increased muscle activity in pericranial muscles, and (2) those not associated with increased muscle activity.

The relationship between tension-type headache, the myofascial pain syndrome, and fibromyalgia is complex. Myofascial nociception coupled with abnormal central modulation of this information may produce the central dysfunction that results in tension-type headache. This may involve ascending and descending pain-modulating pathways, the cortex, the limbic system, the thalamus, and the brain stem.

Although the role of muscles in causing tension-type headache is fairly evident, the central brain and brain stem factors involved in migraine are less obvious. As migraine and tension-type headache are closely related clinically and may overlap in some patients, it is realistic to expect some of the neurovascular changes of migraine to be operative in severe cases of tension-type headache.

Some researchers believe that there is a continuum, in which patients who exhibit migraine with aura are at one end of the spectrum and patients with simple tension-type headaches are at the other, sharing a similar pathophysiology.

Mathew and coworkers (1987) have shown that most adults with chronic tension-type headache had migraine at earlier ages, then **transformed** to a mixed headache pattern known as *chronic daily headache*. Thus, there is some justification for the assumption that the pathophysiology of the two conditions may be similar or even identical.

The Pathophysiology of Cluster Headache

Cluster headache was first described by Romberg and Eulenburg in the middle and late 19th century, respectively. It became well known after Horton and associates described it in 1939, concluding that cluster headache is due to intrinsic histamine-mediated dilation of the external carotid artery. Ekbom reported its periodic nature in 1947. In 1952, Kunkle and colleagues focused attention on the salient characteristic of cluster headache and suggested the term "headache in cluster pattern."

In the 1970s, investigators focused on a search for pathology in the internal carotid artery because retro-orbital pain suggested such a location. Kudrow (1980) found decreased supraorbital artery flow velocity ipsilateral to the pain on Doppler flow studies as well as decreased temperatures in the supraorbital area on facial thermography. Many researchers have found evidence of impaired sympathetic activity by studying the pupil, the heart, and facial sweating patterns.

BIOCHEMICAL AND HORMONAL DYSFUNCTION

The role of histamine has been extensively investigated and is still unclear. Anthony and Lance (1971) found significantly elevated levels of histamine during headache periods. Appenzeller and coworkers (1981) found evidence of mast cell degranulation in skin biopsies taken from the temporal area in cluster headache patients. They suggested that histamine released from mast cells near cutaneous nerves may cause changes in blood vessel size. Kudrow (1976) found a decrease in plasma testosterone and luteinizing hormone levels in cluster patients during cluster periods. This may not be a problem specific to cluster headache but is possibly related to any pain syndrome that may upset the normal hypothalamic-pituitary-adrenal axis function.

CHRONOBIOLOGICAL ABNORMALITIES

The endocrine changes just mentioned prompted a study of other neuroendocrine functions and their rhythmicity. A change in the circadian (circadian comes from circa-diem, which means approximately 1 day) rhythmicity was reported for multiple neuroendocrine hormones. In 1988, Bussone and associates demonstrated reduced thyrotropin response to thyrotropin-releasing hormone during cluster periods, supporting a putative abnormality of the hypothalamic-pituitary axis in cluster headache. Kudrow postulated that a disturbance of circadian rhythmicity of neuroendocrine substances occurs cyclically because of a circannual (approximately 1 year) periodicity. He further suggested that the pathology may occur in the hypothalamic suprachiasmatic nucleus, the locus of the biological clock.

Many patients report that cluster attacks occur at the same time of the year, usually once or twice each year. Kudrow studied 400 male patients over a 10-year period and recorded the onset of the cluster periods in 891 instances. He found a bimodal curve with peak frequencies of onset in July and January, approximately 2 weeks following the longest and shortest days of the year. The pattern was interrupted briefly during the two weeks following the resetting of clocks for daylight savings time. He concluded that there was an association between cluster period onset and photoperiod changes and postulated that failure of the suprachiasmatic nucleus in the hypothalamus to synchronize with the photoperiods was to blame. This may explain why cluster patients frequently go into a cluster period when they travel rapidly across time zones in a plane or need to change their sleep-wake cycle by getting up or going to sleep at a different time.

In 1959, Kunkle suggested that cluster headache attacks resulted from paroxysmal overactivity of the seventh and tenth cranial nerves. Neurosurgeons have tried sectioning either the greater superficial petrosal nerve or the nervous intermedius and have met with some success in treating cluster patients.

Moskowitz believes that the trigeminovascular system mediates pain in cluster headache. He proposed that the most central site of pathology is the cavernous sinus. Sicuteri and associates (1985) proposed substance P and other neurotransmitters as the media-tors of pain and suggested that somatostatin, an inhibitor of substance P, could alleviate cluster attacks.

THE ROLE OF THE CAROTID BODY AND SLEEP

Lee Kudrow proposed in 1983 that the carotid body, located in the bulb of the carotid artery in the neck, had blunted activity caused by discharges from the hypothalamus. He suggested that this would manifest itself as hypoxemia during sleep. Oxygen desaturation would result, and lack of oxygen to the chemoreceptors in the carotid body would cause impulses to stimulate the medulla and affect respiration and cause pain.

In further studies, Kudrow demonstrated a higher incidence of sleep apnea in cluster patients, which awakened them during rapid eye movement states. Lee and David Kudrow found that nitroglycerin decreased the oxygen saturation in cluster patients during active cluster periods, culminating in a cluster attack. These results confirm the hypothesis that persistent relative hypoxemia, due to impairment of chemoreceptor autoregulation, characterizes the cluster period.

This may explain why most cluster patients can be treated effectively by inhalation of pure oxygen during a cluster attack. Decreased oxygen saturation at high altitudes (over 5000 feet above sea level) often produces cluster attacks; many cluster patients have attacks during airplane travel because cabins are pressurized to approximately 7500 feet above sea level.

Although it is hard to put all of these facts together into a clear hypothesis that explains the origin of cluster headache, the following brief summary of Lee Kudrow's theory is helpful:

The cluster period may involve an altered physiological state of the brain and its connections, characterized by dysfunction in the hypothalamus that results in chronobiological abnormalities and impaired autonomic function. This leads to autoregulatory deficiencies in vasomotor regulation and altered responses of the chemoreceptors in the carotid body to falling oxygen levels. In this state an attack can be provoked by sustained decreased oxygen levels. The brain stem is involved at the level of the pons and medulla as well as the fifth, seventh, ninth, and tenth cranial nerves. Blood vessel changes that may be mediated by several neuropeptides occur, especially in the cavernous sinus.

Conclusion

Since the 17th century, many theories of headache have been proposed. Several of these theories have provided useful bases for further research and positive findings as to the pathophysiology of the primary headache disorders. Current studies suggest that the pathophysiology of migraine and tension-type headaches may be closely related. Taken as a whole, previous and current research provide an ever-growing body of knowledge that has steadily improved the treatment of headache over the past half century and promises to bring major breakthroughs in the next decade.

SUGGESTED READINGS

Aghajanian GH: The modulatory role of serotonin at multiple receptors in brain. In Jacobs BL, Gelperin A, eds, *Serotonin Neurotransmission and Behavior.* Cambridge, MA: MIT Press. 1981;156.

Anthony M, Hinterberger H, Lance JW: The possible relationship of serotonin to the migraine syndrome. *Res Clin Stud Headache.* 1969;2:29.

Anthony M, Hinterberger H, Lance JW: Plasma serotonin in migraine and stress. *Arch Neurol.* 1967;16:544.

Anthony M, Lance JW: Histamine and serotonin in cluster headache. *Arch Neurol.* 1971;25:225.

Appenzeller O, Becker WJ, Ragaz A: Cluster headache: Ultrastructural aspects and pathogenetic mechanisms. *Arch Neurol.* 1981;38:302.

Arregui A, Cabrera J, Leon-Velarde F, et al: High prevalence of migraine in a high altitude population. *Neurology.* 1991;41:1668.

Barkley AL, Tepley N, Nagel-Leiby S, et al: Magnetoencephalographic studies of migraine. *Headache.* 1990;30:428.

Bruyn GW: The biochemistry of migraine. *Headache.* 1980;20:235.

Bussone G, Frediani F, Leone M: TRH test in cluster headache. *Headache.* 1988;28:462.

Buzzi MG, Moskowitz MA: The antimigraine drug Sumatriptan (GR43175) selectively blocks neurogenic plasma extravasation from blood vessels in dura mater. *Br J Pharmacol.* 1990;99:202–206.

Dalessio DJ: *Wolff's Headache and Other Head Pain,* 5th ed. New York: Oxford University Press. 1987.

Drummond PD, Lance JW: Extracranial vascular changes and the source of pain in migraine headache. *Ann Neurol.* 1983;13:32–37.

Edmeads J: Headache: Changing perspectives and controversies. In *Update on headache: A comprehensive course in mechanisms and management,* a study booklet from the Postgraduate Course of the American Association for the Study of Headache, 1991.

Edvinsson L, Degueurce A, MacKenzie ET, et al: Central serotonergic nerves project to the pial vessels of the brain. *Nature.* 1983;306:55–57.

Ekbom K: Nitroglycerin as a provocative agent in cluster headache. *Arch Neurol.* 1968;19:487–493.

Ekbom KA: Ergotamine tartrate orally in Horton's histaminic cephalgia (also called Harris' "ciliary neuralgia"): A new method of treatment. *Acta Psychiatr Scand.* 1947;46(suppl):106.

Eulenburg A: *Lehrbuch der Nervenkrankheiten,* 2nd ed. Vol 2. Berlin: Hirschwald. 1878;264.

Featherstone HJ: Migraine and muscle contraction headache: A continuum. *Headache.* 1985;25:194.

Ferrari MD, Odink J, Tapparelli C, et al: Serotonin metabolism in migraine. *Neurology.* 1989;39:1239–1242.

Fields HL: *Pain: Mechanisms and Management.* New York: McGraw-Hill. 1987.

Gawel M, Burkett M, Rose FC: The platelet release action during a migraine attack. *Headache.* 1979;19:323.

Goadsby PJ, Edvinsson L, Ekman R: Vasoactive peptide release in the extracerebral circulation of the human during migraine headache. *Ann Neurol.* 1990;28:183–187.

Goadsby PJ, Gundlach AL: Localization of 3H-dihydroergotamine-binding sites in the cat central nervous system: Relevance to migraine. *Ann Neurol.* 1991;29:91.

Goadsby PJ, Zagami AS, Lambert GA: Neural processing of craniovascular pain: A synthesis of the central structures involved in migraine. *Headache.* 1991;31:365.

Graham JR, Wolff HG: Mechanisms of migraine headache and action of ergotamine tartrate. *Arch Neurol Psychiatry.* 1938;39:737–763.

Greden JF, Victor BS, Fontaine P, et al: Caffeine withdrawal headache: A clinical profile. *Psychodynamics.* 1980;21:411.

Hanington E: The platelet and migraine. *Headache.* 1986;26:411.

Henderson WR, Raskin NH: "Hot-dog" headache: Individual susceptibility to nitrite. *Lancet.* 1972;2:1162–1163.

Hilton BP, Cummings JN: An assessment of platelet aggregation induced by 5-hydroxytryptamine. *J Clin Pathol.* 1971;24:250.

Horton BT: Histaminic cephalalgia. *Lancet.* 1952;2:92–98.

Horton BT, MacLean AR, Craig WM: A new syndrome of vascular headache: Results of treatment with histamine. Preliminary report. *Mayo Clin Proc.* 1939;14:257.

Johnson ES: A basis for migraine therapy: The autonomic theory reappraised. *Postgrad Med J.* 1978;54:231.

Joutel A, Bousser MG, Biousse V, et al: A gene for familial hemiplegic migraine maps to chromosome 19. *Nat Genet.* 1993;5:40–45.

Koehler SM, Glaros A: The effect of aspartame on migraine headache. *Headache.* 1988;28:10.

Kudrow L: A possible role of the carotid body in the pathogenesis of cluster headache. *Cephalalgia.* 1983;3:241–247.

Kudrow L: Response of cluster headache attacks to oxygen inhalation. *Headache.* 1981;21:1–4.

Kudrow L: *Cluster Headache: Mechanisms and Management,* 4th ed. London: Oxford University Press. 1980.

Kudrow L: Plasma testosterone levels in cluster headache: Preliminary results. *Headache.* 1976;16:28–31.

Kudrow L: The relationship of headache frequency to hormonal use in migraine. *Headache.* 1975;15:36.

Kudrow L, Kudrow DB: Association of sustained oxyhemoglobin desaturation and onset of cluster headache attacks. *Headache.* 1990;30:474–480.

Kudrow L, McGinty DJ, Phillips ER, et al: Sleep apnea in cluster headache. Proceedings of the 12th Scandinavian Migraine Society Meeting, Helsinki, June 17–18. 1984, p. 56.

Kunkle EC, Pfeiffer JB Jr, Wilhoit WM, et al: Recurrent brief headache in "cluster" pattern. *Trans Am Neurol Assoc.* 1952;77:240.

Lance JW: A concept of migraine and the search for the ideal headache drug. *Headache.* 1990;30(Suppl 1):17.

Lance JW: *Mechanisms and Management of Headache,* 4th ed. London: Butterworth Publications. 1982.

Lance JW, Lambert GA, Zagami AS: 5-Hydroxytryptamine and its putative etiological involvement in migraine. *Cephalalgia.* 1989;9(Suppl 9):7.

Lauritzen M: Pathophysiology of the migraine aura: The spreading depression theory. *Brain.* 1994;117:199–210.

Leão AAP: Spreading depression of activity in cerebral cortex. *J Neurophysiol.* 1944;7:359–390.

Marrelli A, Marini C, Principe M: Seasonal and meteorological factors in primary headaches. *Headache.* 1988;28:111.

Mathew NT, Reuveni NT, Perez F: Transformed or evolutive migraine. *Headache.* 1987;27:102.

Mayberg MR, Zervas NT, Moskowitz MA: Trigeminal projections to supratentorial pial and dural blood vessels in cats demonstrated by horseradish peroxidase histochemistry. *J Comp Neurol.* 1984;223:46–56.

Medina JL, Diamond SD: The role of diet in migraine. *Headache.* 1978;18:31.

Milner PM: Note on a possible correspondence between scotomas of migraine and spreading depression of Leão. *Electroencephalogr Clin Neurophysiol.* 1958; 10:705.

Moskowitz MA: Basic mechanisms in vascular headache. *Neurol Clin.* 1990;8:801.

Moskowitz MA: Neurology of vascular head pain. *Ann Neurol.* 1984;33:335.

Olesen J, Larsen B, Lauritzen M: Focal hyperemia followed by spreading oligemia and impaired activation of rCBF in classic migraine. *Ann Neurol.* 1981;9:344–352.

Olesen J: Vascular aspects of migraine pathophysiology. In Rose FC, ed, *Proceedings of the 5th International Migraine Symposium, London, 1984.* Basel: Karger. 1985;130.

Penfield W, McHaughton F: Dural headache and innervation of the dura mater. *Arch Neurol Psychiatry.* 1940;44:43.

Rapport MM: Serum vasoconstrictor (serotonin). V: The presence of creatinine in the complex. A proposed structure of the vasoconstrictor principle. *J Biol Chem.* 1949;180:961.

Raskin NH: On the origin of head pain. *Headache.* 1988;28:254.

Raskin NH: Serotonin receptors and headache. *N Engl J Med.* 1991;325:353.

Raskin NH, Hosobuchi Y, Lamb S: Headache may arise from perturbation of brain. *Headache.* 1987;27:416.

Ray BS, Wolff HG: Experimental studies in headache: Pain sensitive structures of the head and their significance in headache. *Arch Surg.* 1940;41:813.

Romberg MH: *Lehrbuch der Nervenkrankheiten des Menschen,* Band I. Berlin: Dunker. 1840;58.

Sacks O: *Migraine: Understanding a Common Disorder.* Berkeley and Los Angeles: University of California Press. 1985.

Sainsbury P, Gibson JG: Symptoms of anxiety and tension and the accompanying physiological changes in the muscular system. *J Neurol Neurosurg Psychiatry.* 1954;17:216.

Saito K, Markowitz S, Moskowitz MA: Ergot alkaloids block neurogenic extravasation in dura mater: Proposed action in vascular headaches. *Ann Neurol.* 1988;24:732.

Sakai F, Meyer JS: Abnormal cerebrovascular reactivity in patients with migraine and cluster headache. *Headache.* 1979;23:284.

Schaumburg H. Chinese-restaurant syndrome. *N Engl J Med.* 1968;278:1122.

Schmidt AW, Peroutka SJ: 5-Hydroxytriptamine receptor families. *FASEB J.* 1989;3:2242.

Scopp AL: MSG and hydrolyzed vegetable protein–induced headache: Review and case studies. *Headache.* 1991;31:107.

Sicuteri F: Endorphins, opiate receptors and migraine headache. *Headache.* 1978;17:253.

Sicuteri F, Boccuni M, Fanciullacci M, et al: Naloxone effectiveness of spontaneous and induced perceptive disorders in migraine. *Headache.* 1983;23:179.

Sicuteri F, Fanciullacci M, Geppetti P, et al: Substance-P mechanism in cluster headache: Evaluation in plasma and cerebrospinal fluid. *Cephalalgia.* 1985; 5:143.

Sicuteri F, Testi A, Anselmi B: Biochemical investigations in headache: Increase in hydroxyindolacetic acid excretion during migraine attacks. *Int Arch Allergy Immunol.* 1961;19:55.

Silberstein SD, Merriam MD: Estrogens, progestins, and headache. *Neurology.* 1991;41:786.

Sjaastad O: Chronic paroxysmal hemicrania: Clinical aspects and controversies. In Blau JN, ed, *Migraine: Clinical, Therapeutic, Conceptual and Research Aspects.* London: Chapman and Hall. 1987;135–152.

Sjaastad, O: *Cluster Headache Syndrome.* London: W. B. Saunders. 1992.

Sjaastad O, Dale I: Evidence for a new (?) treatable headache entity. *Headache.* 1974;14:105–108.

Skyhøj-Olsen T, Friberg L, Lassen NA: Ischemia may be the primary cause of the neurologic deficits in classic migraine. *Arch Neurol.* 1987;44:156–161.

Smith RO: Ice cream headache. In Vinken PJ, Bruyn GW, eds, *Headaches and Cranial Neuralgias. (Handbook of Clinical Neurology, vol 5.)* Amsterdam: North-Holland Publishing. 1968;188.

Somerville BW: The role of progesterone and estradiol upon migraine. *Headache.* 1972;12:93.

Tunis MM, Wolff HG: Studies on headache: Long-term observations of the reactivity of the cranial arteries in subjects with vascular headache of the migraine type. *Arch Neurol Psychiatry.* 1953;70:551.

Welch KMA: Migraine: A biobehavioral disorder. *Arch Neurol.* 1987;44:323.

Welch KMA, D'Andrea A, Tepley N, et al: The concept of migraine as a state of central neuronal hyperexcitability. *Neurol Clin.* 1990;8:817.

Wolf HG: *Headache and Other Head Pain,* 2nd ed. New York: Oxford University Press. 1963.

Woods RP, Iacoboni M, Mazziotta JC: Brief report: Bilateral spreading cerebral hypoperfusion during spontaneous migraine headache. *N Engl J Med.* 1995; 331:1689.

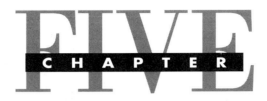

The History and Physical Examination

Setting the Tone

A complete and accurate history is the most important aspect of any initial consultation, and in particular those for headache. In over 90% of cases, the history will establish the diagnosis or lead to a differential diagnosis, which may be further clarified by examination and diagnostic testing when necessary.

History taking is the first step in establishing a patient-physician alliance that is based on mutual respect and trust. Headache patients not only want headache relief, they also seek physicians who are genuinely concerned about their well-being and who project a positive attitude. Skepticism, disbelief, and an adversarial manner are counterproductive and have the potential to completely disrupt the physician-patient relationship.

Physicians should be keenly aware of their own attitudes about headache patients The two most extreme ends of these beliefs are 1) that patients are neurotic sufferers or 2) they suffer from a neurobiological disorder. Pain is a complex phenomenon that may be influenced by neurological, physiological, biochemical, genetic, psychological, and sociocultural factors. Pain must be understood in the context of the human experi-ence; thus, patients with the same symptom complex may react differently to pain.

Clinicians should always be mindful of the following three rules:

1 Patients are to be believed, and it is important to address their questions.
2 Patients' complaints should be accepted and investigated.
3 Clinicians must display interest, empathy, and concern.

The intensity of the pain and the effect on the patient's life should be viewed in an atmosphere of compassion and credibility. Enough time should be set aside for the initial consultation; this time should allow for the history, examination, patient questions, the physician's answers and explanations, and patient education, which will be discussed in detail in Chapter 7.

The History

The headache history should include the following major areas:
1) Age of Onset and Description of Early Headache
2) Frequency
   a) Previous

b) Current
c) Mode of increase, gradual or sudden
3) Location of Pain
4) Description of Pain
5) Duration of Pain
6) Description of the Prodrome
7) Description of the Aura
8) Associated Symptoms
9) Behavior During Headache
10) Trigger Factors
11) Past Medications (including nonprescription medications)
    a) Types (brand or generic)
    b) Dosages
    c) Frequency of administration
    d) Duration of administration and dates
    e) Routes of administration
    f) Effectiveness
    g) Side effects
    h) Allergies
12) Current Medications (for headache and other conditions)
13) Past Medical History
14) Past Surgical History
15) Family History (especially of headache)
16) Habit History (including sleep, smoking, and alcohol/drugs)
17) Menstrual History and Hormonal Factors
18) Psychosocial History
19) Diagnosis

Figures 5–1 and 5–2 show a set of the forms we use in gathering patient histories. We have found it helpful to have patients fill out the forms in Figure 5–1 prior to the first visit. Once the patient is in the office, these forms are reviewed and amplified as necessary before being summarized on a face sheet as shown in Figure 5–3. Our summary face sheet is a modification of one suggested by Dr. Lee Kudrow of The California Medical Clinic for Headache in Encino, California. Following the format used for our headache calendars, we rate headache intensities on a 4-point scale from 0 to 3. We then take a detailed history for each level of intensity. A number 3 headache refers to extreme severity or total incapacitation. A number 2 headache refers to moderate pain that is significant but not incapacitating. A number 1 headache is characterized by mild

pain that does not interfere with function and is often experienced as a dull background sense of being less than clear-headed when attention is not focused elsewhere.

Working with this model, we generally find that migraine and cluster headache fall in the more severe (2 and 3) categories, whereas tension-type headache usually is characterized by number 1 intensity and occasionally by number 2.

We find it important to go through the parameters of the headache history for each level of intensity. After completing our questions, patients are asked to add anything we may not have included. This format of history-taking facilitates exposure of different types of headache and differentiates them by intensity, location, pain quality, and a variety of associated symptoms.

Let us now go through the history step by step using the format presented on the summary face sheet in Figure 5–3. We will evaluate the history for each level of intensity in order to distinguish headache types from one another. Please see the patient information and medical history forms in Figure 5–1. These forms provide space in which to record in detail all current and past medications, headache triggers, medical history, surgical history, family history, habit history, sleep history, allergies, diagnostic tests, non-medication treatments, and a general overview of psychosocial and psychological factors.

Having patients fill out these forms before coming to the initial consultation saves time and improves accuracy, but the forms can also be filled out when patients present for the initial visit. A nurse or physician can summarize all critical factors to give a concise, comprehensive overview.

We generally start by reviewing the parameters described for the most severe headaches, then we cover moderate and dull intensities, in that order. There is space in which to summarize demographic data on the summary face sheet, and this information is of paramount importance. Occupational factors such as being in fixed postural positions for long periods of time, exposure to environmental triggers, and hours of work

Text continued on page 67

The New England Center for Headache

Date of First Visit _____

First Name _____ M.I. _____ Last Name _____

Marital Status ☐ Married ☐ Single ☐ Separated ☐ Widowed ☐ Divorced

Birthdate _____ Age _____ Sex M _____ F _____

Patient's SS # _____-_____-_____

Spouse's First Name _____ M.I. _____ Last Name _____

Spouse's SS # _____-_____-_____

Spouse's Birthdate _____ Age _____ Sex M _____ F _____

Address _____ City _____ State _____ Zip _____

Home Phone ( ) _____ Work Phone ( ) _____ Extension _____ Fax ( ) _____

****

Occupation _____

Employed By _____

Address _____ City _____ State _____ Zip _____

Insurance Company _____

Address _____ City _____ State _____ Zip _____

Policy Number # _____ Group # _____ Phone ( ) _____

Spouse's Occupation _____

Employed By _____

Address _____ City _____ State _____ Zip _____

Work Phone ( ) _____

Insurance Company _____

Address _____ City _____ State _____ Zip _____

Policy Number # _____ Group # _____ Phone ( ) _____

IF PATIENT IS UNDER 18 YEARS PLEASE INCLUDE THE FOLLOWING:

Parent's/Guardian's Name _____
(Person who is guarantor for the bill)

Address _____ City _____ State _____ Zip _____

Home Phone ( ) _____ Work Phone ( ) _____

Social Security # _____-_____-_____ Birthdate _____

Who is your personal physician? _____ Specialty? _____

Address _____ City _____ State _____ Zip _____

Phone ( ) _____ Fax ( ) _____

How did you hear about The New England Center for Headache? _____

Do you want a letter sent to any doctor? ☐ YES ☐ NO

Address _____ City _____ State _____ Zip _____

Letter dictated to _____ Date _____

(For office use only)

Figure 5–1

Patient information and medical history forms to be filled out by the patient before the initial visit. This is placed on the inside of the front cover of the chart.

Illustration continued on following page

The New England Center for Headache
778 Long Ridge Road • Stamford, CT 06902-1249 • Phone (203) 968-1799
FAX (203) 968-8303

**PATIENT INFORMATION
AND
MEDICAL HISTORY**

INSTRUCTIONS: Please complete the information below and on the following pages. If you are not certain about how to answer a particular question, leave it blank and we will discuss it when you come in. It is important that you answer as completely as possible. Our goal is your wellness. To achieve it, we need to know all about you.

HEADACHE AND OTHER MEDICATIONS

Please list <u>*ALL CURRENT*</u> medications (headache first then other) you are taking, including aspirin, Tylenol, birth control pills, hormones, vitamins, cold and sinus pills, sleeping pills, etc.

ALL *CURRENT* MEDICATIONS YOU ARE TAKING
First preventive medications then abortive (Use the back of this page if necessary)

Name of Medication	Dose in mg per pill	How taken (pill, patch, suppository)	# Times taken per day	How long taken (wks or mos)	Year	Relief* (0–3)	Side effects?

PREVIOUS HEADACHE MEDICATIONS YOU HAVE TAKEN
First preventive medications then abortive (Use the back of this page if necessary)

Name of Medication	Dose in mg per pill	How taken (pill, patch, suppository)	# Times taken per day	How long taken (wks or mos)	Year	Relief* (0–3)	Side effects?

*RELIEF CODE: 0 = NO RELIEF   1 = MILD RELIEF   2 = MODERATE RELIEF   3 = COMPLETE RELIEF

Figure 5–1

Continued.

ALL CURRENT MEDICATIONS YOU ARE TAKING (Continued)
First preventive medications then abortive

Name of Medication	Dose in mg per pill	How taken (pill, patch, suppository)	# Times taken per day	How long taken (wks or mos)	Year	Relief* (0–3)	Side effects?

PREVIOUS HEADACHE MEDICATIONS YOU HAVE TAKEN (Continued)
First preventive medications then abortive

Name of Medication	Dose in mg per pill	How taken (pill, patch, suppository)	# Times taken per day	How long taken (wks or mos)	Year	Relief* (0–3)	Side effects?

*RELIEF CODE: 0 = NO RELIEF   1 = MILD RELIEF   2 = MODERATE RELIEF   3 = COMPLETE RELIEF

©1995 The New England Center for Headache

Figure 5–1

Continued (back of form).

Illustration continued on following page

The New England Center for Headache

HEADACHE TRIGGERS

Please circle all of the following that you feel may "trigger" or start your severe headaches:

Alcohol	Fasting	Lack of sleep	Sex	Weekends	Vacation
Menses	Foods	Too much sleep	Orgasm	Exertion	Medication
Seasonal	Weather	Allergies/Sinus	Emotions	Stress	Sun
Odors	Altitude	Let down	Bright light	Other	

PAST MEDICAL HISTORY

Date of your last complete physical exam _____

Done by _____

If you have had any of the following health problems, please check the appropriate box, then provide a brief description of the problem and the date the problem occurred.

☐ Accident _____

☐ Trauma to the head or neck _____

☐ Loss of consciousness _____

☐ Episodic vomiting/motion sickness/vertigo _____

☐ High blood pressure _____

☐ Heart disease or Raynaud's disease (white hands in the cold) _____

☐ Ear, nose, throat, or sinus problems _____

☐ Dental and/or TMJ problems _____

☐ Cervical spine problems (neck pain) _____

☐ Thyroid problems _____

☐ Ulcer, irritable bowel, or other GI problems _____

☐ Endometriosis or irregular periods _____

☐ Sexual problems _____

☐ Other _____

HAVE YOU EVER BEEN HOSPITALIZED FOR

☐ Suicide attempt _____

☐ Depression _____

☐ Eating disorder _____

☐ Detoxification _____

☐ Glaucoma _____

☐ Prostate or urinary problems _____

☐ TB, AIDS, or other infection _____

☐ Heart disease _____

☐ Cancer _____

☐ Lung or breathing problems or asthma _____

☐ Other _____

©1995 The New England Center for Headache

Figure 5–1

Continued.

The New England Center for Headache

PAST SURGICAL HISTORY

Please list all surgery you have undergone by the type of operation you had, the date, and where you had it done. Include any problems that developed during or as a result of the surgery.

TYPE	DATE	PLACE
_____	_____	_____
_____	_____	_____
_____	_____	_____
_____	_____	_____

FAMILY HISTORY

Does anyone in your family (grandparents, parents, uncles, aunts, siblings, children) have HEADACHES? If so, who and what type of headache?

_____

_____

Does anyone in your family have NEUROLOGICAL PROBLEMS such as seizures or stroke? If so, who and what type of problem?

_____

_____

Does anyone in your family have INHERITED MEDICAL PROBLEMS? If so, who and what type of problem?

_____

_____

Please check the appropriate box and list which family member has the problem and what specifically that problem is.

☐ Heart problems _____

☐ Psychiatric problems _____

☐ Allergies _____

☐ Women: At what age did your mother go into menopause? _____

HABIT HISTORY

Do you smoke now?   ☐ YES   ☐ NO

  If yes, how many packs per day? _____   How many years have you smoked? _____

  Have you quit smoking? ☐ YES   ☐ NO   If so, when? _____

  How many times have you quit? _____

Do you drink alcohol?   ☐ YES   ☐ NO

  If yes, how often do you drink?   ☐ DAILY ☐ 1–2 TIMES/WEEK ☐ OCCASIONALLY ☐ RARELY

  How much of what each time? _____

  Do you follow a 12 step program? ☐ YES ☐ NO

  When did you quit?

©1995 The New England Center for Headache

Figure 5–1

Continued.

Illustration continued on following page

The New England Center for Headache

Do you drink coffee, tea, or colas? ☐ YES ☐ NO

If you drink coffee, how many cups or mugs do you drink daily of:

Brewed _____ Instant _____ Decaffeinated _____

If you drink tea, how many cups per day? _____ Decaffeinated _____ Caffeinated

If you drink ice tea, how many glasses per day? _____ Decaffeinated _____ Caffeinated

If you drink colas, how many cans/glasses per day? _____ Decaffeinated _____ Caffeinated

SLEEP HISTORY

Do you sleep well? ☐ YES ☐ NO

Do you feel rested most mornings? ☐ YES ☐ NO

Do you awaken during the night? ☐ YES ☐ NO   What time? _____   How many times? _____

How long does it take you to fall asleep? _____

Usual sleep time? _____ Wake time? _____

ALLERGIES

Are you allergic to IVP dye (kidney test) or CT scan dye? ☐ YES ☐ NO

If yes, what reaction do you have? _____

Do you have allergies to medications? ☐ YES ☐ NO

If yes, please list all medications _____

Do you have asthma or emphysema? ☐ YES ☐ NO   Other _____

PREVIOUS EVALUATIONS FOR HEADACHE

TEST	BY WHOM & WHERE?	RESULT or DIAGNOSIS	YEAR
Neurological Consultation			
Headache Specialist			
CT Scan of Brain (with dye?) ☐ YES ☐ NO			
MRI Scan of Brain (with dye?) ☐ YES ☐ NO			
MRI or CT Scan of Neck			
EEG, Evoked Potentials, BAER			
Sinus X-rays or Scan of Sinuses			
Spinal Tap			
Angiogram (Arteriogram)			
Doppler/Thermography			
EKG (Heart)			
Ear, Nose & Throat Consultation			

Continued on next page

©1995 The New England Center for Headache

Figure 5–1

Continued.

The New England Center for Headache

PREVIOUS EVALUATIONS FOR HEADACHE Continued

TEST	BY WHOM & WHERE?	RESULT or DIAGNOSIS	YEAR
TMJ Specialist			
Allergy Testing			
Psychological Testing			
Other Testing			

PREVIOUS TREATMENTS

Please check the appropriate box(es), then list by whom and where you underwent treatment, what the results were, and when.

	BY WHOM & WHERE	DIAGNOSIS?	DID IT HELP?	YEAR
☐ Acupuncture				
☐ Chiropractic				
☐ Nutritional Therapy				
☐ Psychotherapy and/or Behavior Therapy				
☐ Biofeedback				
☐ Self-Hypnosis				
☐ Trigger Point Injections				
☐ Nerve Blocks				
☐ Other				

GENERAL INFORMATION

	ALWAYS	SOMETIMES	NEVER
Are you nervous around strangers?	☐	☐	☐
Do you find it hard to make decisions?	☐	☐	☐
Do you find it hard to concentrate or remember?	☐	☐	☐
Do you feel lonely or depressed?	☐	☐	☐
Do you cry?	☐	☐	☐
Would you say you have a hopeless outlook?	☐	☐	☐
Do you have difficulty relaxing?	☐	☐	☐
Do you have a tendency to worry a great deal?	☐	☐	☐
Are you troubled by dreams or thoughts?	☐	☐	☐
Do you have a tendency to be shy or sensitive?	☐	☐	☐
Do you have a strong dislike of criticism?	☐	☐	☐
Do you lose your temper?	☐	☐	☐
Do minor annoyances make you angry?	☐	☐	☐
Do you become very disturbed by family problems?	☐	☐	☐
Do you become very disturbed by problems at work?	☐	☐	☐
Do you have sexual difficulties?	☐	☐	☐
Have you considered committing suicide?	☐	☐	☐
Are you susceptible to intense feelings of guilt?	☐	☐	☐

Have you ever desired or sought psychiatric help? ☐ YES ☐ NO

Is there a possibility that you may be pregnant? ☐ YES ☐ NO

Please list any problems or factors not listed above that you feel may have something to do with either causing or intensifying your headaches. (You may attach a blank page if needed.)

_____

_____

_____

*Thank you for spending the time on these forms. The information provided will help us to better understand you and your headaches.

Figure 5–1

Continued.

The New England Center for Headache
778 Long Ridge Road • Stamford, Connecticut 06902 • (203) 968-1799
Intake Summary and Treatment Plan

Date	Name			Further Plans
	Age Sex			
	Onset			
	Diagnoses			
	Frequency			
	#3 (severe)	#2 (moderate)	#1 (mild)	
	Neurological Examination			
	MMPI			
	PPP (Psychophysiological Profile)			Laboratory Investigations
				EEG Reason:
	Medication Prescribed			Flash VEP
	Abortive:			P-300
				BAER
				CT of: Place:
				MRI of: Place:
				Reason:
	Preventive:			Bloods: CBC ESR LFT LYME
				GCP, TSH Drug Screen
				Levels: Depakote, DPH, Tegretol; Amitrip; Nortrip
	Behavioral Treatment Plan:			Other:
	Calendar			
	Elimination Diet			
	Biofeedback			
	Exercise Program			
	Vitamins, minerals			
	Other			

©1991 The New England Center for Headache

Figure 5–2

Physician's summary sheet.

The New England Center for Headache
778 Long Ridge Road • Stamford, Connecticut 06902 • (203) 968-1799

REVISIT SHEET   RV _____   PC _____
(phone conference)

Name: _____ Date: _____ Page: _____

Status   ☐ Improved   ☐ Stable   ☐ Deteriorated

Problems: _____
_____
_____
_____
_____
_____

Preventive Medications   Problems
_____   _____
_____   _____
_____   _____
_____   _____
_____   _____

Headache Frequency (per month)   Abortive Medications   Problems

Month	#3	#2	#1

(Baseline Frequencies)

Other Medications

Total number of days of work missed and/or dysfunctional: _____   Days since last RV: _____

Number of days of work missed: _____   Number of acute care visits: _____

Number of days greater than 50% dysfunctional: _____   Number of acute care phone contacts at NECH: _____

Plan _____
_____
_____
_____
_____

RV \   Weeks   Months   Annual
PC /

Provider: _____

Figure 5–2
Continued.

The New England Center for Headache
778 Long Ridge Road • Stamford, CT 06902 • (203) 968-1799
Face Sheet

Name: _____ Date: _____ Ref: _____
                                                                                                    (referred by)

Age: _____ Sex: _____ Marital Status: S   M   SEP   D   W

Intensity:	Severe (3)	Moderate (2)	Dull (1)	Menstrual & Hormonal History

Onset

Frequency ⎡—Previous
         ⎣—Current

Habits:
(alcohol, tobacco, caffeine, sleep, drugs)

Location: R   L   B   A

Description

Medical   Surgical

Duration: Min. Av. Max.   Min. Av. Max.   Min. Av. Max.   Trauma   LOC   S.D.

Prodrome

Aura

Associations: N V A D
Stuffed/Running   dizzy
red/tearing   sono
ptosis/miosis   photo

Psychosocial:

Worse with Exertion

Behavior

Other:

Diagnosis

Current Medication	Previous

Previous Tests:

Figure 5–3
Summary face sheet for the patient information and medical history forms.

(especially those that involve shift change) may provide important clues in relationship to trigger factors.

ONSET

The age of headache onset is important from a number of perspectives. It provides information as to whether the headaches are of recent origin or have been present over a number of years, and it helps to reveal any changes in headache patterns. For example, although chronic headache may have been present for a number of years, the headache may have changed in intensity, quality, location of pain, etc., in such ways as to raise suspicion of organic pathology.

Patients with frequent or severe headaches that begin after the age of 50 should be scrutinized for potential organic causes such as brain tumor or temporal arteritis, particularly in the presence of associated symptoms such as arthralgia, myalgia, loss of vision, and neurological symptoms.

A painful, injected eye with orbital or diffuse pain suggests glaucoma. General guidelines for age of onset of the primary headache disorders are as follows:

Migraine. Migraine onset is typically between 6 and 25 years of age. Bille's studies demonstrated that approximately 5% of children had experienced migraine by the age of 15. The prevalence of migraine prior to puberty is approximately equal in boys and girls, but after puberty, it is almost three times more prevalent in girls than in boys. The American Migraine Study (Lipton et al, 1994) showed that this gender-ratio increases from menarche to about age 42 and then begins to decline but does not equalize, which suggests that more than hormonal factors may be involved in these differences.

Tension-Type Headache. Tension-type headache may occur at any age but is not usually identified by patients as a significant problem until the 20s or 30s.

Cluster Headache. The onset of cluster headache is often in the 30s or 40s.

FREQUENCY AND TIMING

We find it helpful for each level of intensity to review both previous and current frequencies of occurrence. Tertiary care headache centers commonly see patients whose headaches have gradually increased in frequency over a period of years.

Migraine. The frequency of migraine may vary tremendously from once in a lifetime to several attacks per week in its most severe form. The average is one to two attacks per month. The menstrual and hormonal histories often reveal correlations between hormonal events and headache.

Tension-Type Headache. The frequency of tension-type headache varies from occasional to daily; the headache often begins in the late morning or early afternoon.

Cluster Headache. In its episodic or intermittent form, cluster headache may occur over a period of 6 to 8 weeks, with one to two attacks or more during each 24-hour period. Patients with cluster headache are often awakened 60 to 90 minutes after onset of sleep or in the middle of the night. In contrast, migraine headaches are more likely to occur upon awakening at the usual time in the morning. There are no significant periods of remission in the chronic form of cluster headache.

LOCATION OF PAIN

On our summary face sheet, the letters R, L, B, and A represent right, left, bilateral, or alternating. Headaches that match one of these categories are easier to diagnose.

Migraine. The location of migraine may be variable but is often in or behind the eye or in the frontotemporal area. Various studies show a slight predominance of unilateral over bilateral locations. Although the word *migraine* is derived from the Greek word *hemikrania*, migraine pain need not be unilateral and may indeed be holocranial. The location of the pain can vary in an individual patient. Many patients with unilateral headache notice that the pain switches sides from one episode to the next. Headaches that alternate sides are much less likely to be caused by space-occupying lesions.

Tension-Type Headache. Tension-type headaches are most always bilateral and may involve frontal, temporal, parietal, vertex, and occipital areas. They are unilateral approximately 20% of the time. When exclusively unilateral and constant, they fall into the category of *hemicrania continua.*

Cluster Headache. Cluster headache is 100% unilateral in location and most often involves the same side during an attack period. In rare instances, however, the headache may switch sides during an episode or may be on different sides in different episodes. The pain is almost always orbitotemporal in distribution, but it may also involve the maxillary division of the fifth cranial nerve (V_2), the parietal area, or the neck.

DESCRIPTION OF PAIN

Although most patients can describe the quality of their pain, some cannot and may benefit from reviewing a list of pain descriptors.

Migraine. Migraine is more often described as throbbing or pounding, usually in cadence with the pulse. It may also be described as an intense squeezing or pressure from inside the head as though the head might explode, without throbbing.

Tension-Type Headache. The pain of tension-type headache is often described as squeezing, aching, or a sensation or fullness; at times patients report a band-like sensation of pressure around the head as though wearing a tight cap.

Cluster Headache. Patients usually describe cluster pain as excruciating, deep, sharp, boring, relentless pressure from within the skull. In addition, some patients report feeling as though a hot poker is being thrust into an eye and twirled or as though intense pressure from within the skull is pushing an eye outward.

DURATION OF PAIN

Headache duration often provides important diagnostic information. Although variable, the following general guidelines are helpful:

Migraine. Migraine duration may be from 4 to 72 hours. Duration of more than 72 hours is generally associated with medication overuse and rebound phenomena. The average is 12 to 24 hours of intense pain, followed by a period of milder pain that may last as long as 24 hours. In children and in patients who have migraine with aura, the pain typically lasts less than 12 hours.

Tension-Type Headache. Episodic tension-type headache may last from one to several hours, although the International Headache Society (IHS) criteria allow up to 7 days. (See Chap. 2 for a full description of the IHS classification.) In its chronic form, tension-type headache may last from months to years and is most often constant, waxing and waning throughout the day.

Cluster Headache. Individual attacks of cluster headache may last from 30 minutes to 2 hours, with an average duration of 45 to 60 minutes.

PRODROME AND AURA

Migraine. Prodromal symptoms occur in about 30% and aura occurs in 10% to 15% of migraineurs. *Aura* is a transient neurological dysfunction, usually visual, that occurs within 60 minutes before or after headache onset. Visual symptoms include fortification scotomata, photopsias, and blinking or shimmering colored lights that often move slowly across the visual field.

A typical aura does not last more than 20 to 30 minutes and never more than 60 minutes. Prolonged auras may signal more ominous pathology, such as transient ischemic attacks, impending stroke, or an arteriovenous malformation.

Although some patients with migraine with aura, or classic migraine, have the most dramatic symptoms just prior to headache onset, many other patients with migraine notice less specific *prodromal symptoms* for hours before the headache actually begins. Note, however, that most patients with migraine with aura also have migraines without aura.

Prodromal symptoms of migraine are more vague and may involve changes in mood such as elation, depression, and anxiety, as well as fatigue, yawning, and increased urination. Blau (1990) has described these prodromal symptoms and ascribes them to changes in the hypothalamus, suggesting that migraine begins as a central rather than a peripheral process.

Tension-Type Headache. No prodromal symptoms or aura occur.

Cluster. Although prodrome and aura are not usually associated with cluster headache, some patients describe a minor burning sensation in the inner canthus of the eye or the nasal mucosa on the ipsilateral side just prior to the onset of pain.

ASSOCIATED SYMPTOMS

Associated symptoms are very helpful in making the diagnosis of both primary and secondary headache disorders. The symptoms listed on our summary face sheet are more often associated with *primary* rather than secondary headache disorders. The letters N, V, A, and D stand for nausea, vomiting, anorexia, and diarrhea. When considering the possibility of headaches of *organic* origin, particularly when they are of recent onset and associated with symptoms such as fever, myalgia, arthralgia, neurological deficits, neck pain, stuffed nostrils with purulent discharge, and jaw pain, one should think of temporal arteritis, meningitis, structural brain pathology, sinus disease, glaucoma, or temporomandibular joint dysfunction.

Migraine. Symptoms often associated with migraine include nausea, vomiting, anorexia, diarrhea, dizziness, coldness, worsening with activity, and sensitivity to light and sound. Although usually associated with cluster headache, ptosis, miosis, conjunctival injection, lacrimation, and stuffed nostril or running nostril may occur as well.

Tension-Type Headache. Although one does not generally think of associated symp-

toms with tension-type headache, there may be some. In episodic tension-type headache, IHS criteria preclude the presence of nausea or vomiting, although loss of appetite may occur. Patients with episodic tension-type headache may exhibit either photophobia or phonophobia, but not both. (The IHS criteria for migraine states that both must be present.)

Interestingly, in chronic tension-type headache, only one of the following symptoms may be present: photophobia, phonophobia, and nausea. Nausea may be present only if photophobia and phonophobia are absent. If nausea as well as photophobia or phonophobia is present, a diagnosis of migraine must be considered.

Cluster Headache. Associated symptoms may include a partial Horner's syndrome, such as ipsilateral ptosis and miosis, as well as ipsilateral conjunctival injection, and lacrimation. Many patients observe that the ipsilateral nostril becomes stuffed, and as the attack dissipates, it discharges a clear fluid. Nausea and vomiting are generally **not** associated with cluster headache.

BEHAVIOR DURING HEADACHE

Behavior during the headache is a very important criterion in establishing the diagnosis. To document the impact of pain intensity on function, we rate patients' functional ability between 0 and 100%; 0% represents total incapacitation, and 100% represents full and unencumbered functional capacity.

Migraine. The typical behavior of migraine patients is to hibernate or retreat to a dark, quiet room with minimal or no sensory stimuli, to assume a recumbent position, and to sleep if possible. Migraine patients generally state that even mild physical activity during an attack can dramatically increase the pain. Thus, activity such as climbing stairs, bending, or even walking can be a problem. Even when attacks are less than incapacitating, we find that migraine interferes with functional capacity at a greater than 50% level.

Tension-Type Headache. Behavior is generally not affected dramatically with tension-type headache, although there may be a reduction in functional capacity at dull or moderate intensities up to 50% and generally not greater. Activity does not usually worsen the pain, and in fact exercise may ameliorate it. (Note, in contrast, that exercise is likely to worsen migraine pain.)

Cluster Headache. Behavior during cluster headache is strikingly different from that associated with migraine. Generally, patients with cluster headache behave frenetically, as their pain is more intense when they are motionless. They cannot stay still, but pace, rock, drive fists into their eyes or temples, and even bang their heads on a floor or wall.

HABIT HISTORY

We suggest that you summarize the usual habit history of smoking and alcohol and drug use, remembering to include caffeine intake. Excessive use of caffeine can exacerbate migraine in predisposed individuals. In taking a history of coffee intake ask, "cups or mugs" and "decaf or regular." Sleep patterns, including difficulties with sleep onset or sleep maintenance, can be noted here.

MEDICAL-SURGICAL HISTORY

Attention to the details of head trauma is obviously important in establishing a diagnosis of post-traumatic headache and post–head trauma syndrome. Episodes of loss of consciousness or the presence of seizure disorders should also be noted here. You might pay particular attention as to whether or not women have undergone hysterectomy and whether that hysterectomy was partial (one or two ovaries remain) or complete. The presence of comorbid medical problems such as asthma, cardiovascular disorders, and gastrointestinal problems will help you to assess the appropriateness of medications such as β-blockers, vasoconstrictive agents, and nonsteroidal anti-inflammatory medications to make certain there are no contraindications.

MENSTRUAL AND HORMONAL HISTORY

The menstrual and hormonal section of the summary face sheet should include age of menarche, previous or current use of oral contraceptives, and relationship of hormonal fluctuations and events to headache. In this space, you should also include relationship of headache to the menstrual cycle with specific inquiries as to the timing of headache associated with menses or ovulation. In addition, for perimenopausal or postmenopausal women, include the type and manner of estrogen replacement therapy, noting whether that replacement is cyclical or noncyclical and its effect on headache.

As stated in Chapter 4 on pathophysiology, cyclical replacement of estrogen and progesterone may increase migraine frequency. You might also ask about and note any subtle changes in menstrual cycles, such as changes in regularity of the cycle, changes in duration or quantity of flow, and so on, since we often find that even subtle changes may influence migraine frequency and should not be overlooked. Gravida and para frequencies should be included in this section as well.

PSYCHOSOCIAL HISTORY

An essential aspect of history-taking is the psychosocial history. By the time you complete the history and the examination, you should not only have a good idea of whether you are dealing with a primary or secondary headache disorder, you should also have a strong impression about your patient as a person. Pay attention to the effect of headache on *quality of life*. You might find it helpful to ask patients to describe a typical day from the time they awaken until they retire. This should help you to understand your patient's life-style and the possible roles of psychological factors. Specific details related to psychiatric factors and headaches will be covered in Chapter 8. You are looking for a general assessment of your patients at home, at work, and at play. Finally, it is helpful to review the usual symptoms for the presence of *comorbid disorders* such as depression or anxiety which must—if present—be taken into account as part of an overall treatment plan. When you have completed your history taking, be sure to ask if your patients have anything to add or whether there are issues they would like to address.

SUMMARY OF INFORMATION

All previous and current medications as provided on the patient information and medical history forms can be summarized on the summary face sheet. **Do not forget to ask about nonprescription medications in the history.** Tests can be summarized at the bottom of the sheet. The family tree or genogram in the lower right hand corner provides a format in which to summarize relevant family medical history as well as family history of headache, marital relationships, children, and so on. Your review of this summary face sheet will help you make an accurate diagnosis as well as begin to formulate a treatment plan.

Your time is important. As you become more familiar with this history-taking format, you will find that you can obtain an accurate history and formulate a diagnosis in less time than before. Nat Blau, a renowned headache specialist from London, has suggested that some physicians might prefer to use a shortened history format that entails asking 15 questions. The following is a summary of Dr. Blau's suggested headache history:

1) How long have you had this pain?
2) How often does the pain occur?
3) How long does the pain last?
4) Where does the pain begin?
5) Does the pain move around?
6) Is the pain a deep pain, like an ache, or near the surface?
7) What brings on the attacks?
8) What increases the pain or makes it worse?
9) What relieves the pain?
10) What is the pain like?
11) How bad is the pain in terms of affecting daily activities?

12) What else do you notice when you have the pain?
13) What previous treatments have you had?
14) What do you think is the cause of your pain?
15) What brings you to treatment at this time?

We suggest that you might start the history as we originally outlined, using the summary face sheet as a work sheet if you wish. As you become more familiar with the salient aspects of history-taking, you might choose to use Blau's shortened format.

A summary of the different presentations of the primary headache disorders using the parameters outlined in our summary face sheet is shown in Table 5–1.

The Examination

A thorough physical and neurological examination should be conducted following the history (Fig. 5–4). We will outline the more important aspects of the examination, particularly in regard to the complaint of headache. Vital signs should be taken and recorded. Note the general presentation. Does the patient appear to be in pain? Does he or she look sad or tired? Are there physical signs of anxiety such as restlessness, pressured speech, fidgetiness? Does the patient make appropriate eye contact? Is the patient open to your inquiries or is he or she defensive? Open-ended questions about these behaviors are better than statements that might appear confrontational or accusatory. Once general observations are made and recorded, the formal aspects of the examination may begin.

THE HEAD AND NECK

Observe the size and shape of the head, checking for any signs of deformity, unusual bumps or scars. Head circumference should be measured in children to rule out hydrocephalus. Look for ptosis, exophthalmos, asymmetrical pupils, conjunctival injection, and strabismus.

Table 5-1
PRESENTING CHARACTERISTICS OF PRIMARY HEADACHE DISORDERS

	Migraine	Cluster	Tension-Type
Onset	Peak incidence in adolescence	30s or 40s	Variable, generally peak incidence 20s to 40s
Frequency	1 to 2 attacks per month, often with menses; occasionally 4 per month	1 or more attacks per day for 6 to 8 weeks (episodic); several attacks per week without remission (chronic).	Episodic type: less than 15 days per month Chronic type: more than 15 days per month
Location	Unilateral or bilateral; frontotemporal or orbital	100% unilateral; generally orbitotemporal	Bifrontal; biocciptal, neck, shoulders, band-like; infrequently unilateral
Description	Throbbing or intense pressure	Nonthrobbing, excruciating, boring, penetrating	Squeezing, pressing, aching
Duration	4 to 72 hours, usually 12–24 hours	30 minutes to 2 hours, usually 45 to 90 minutes	Episodic type: several hours Chronic type: all day, waxing and waning
Prodrome	Changes in mood, energy, appetite	May include brief mild burning in ipsilateral inner canthus or internal nares	None
Aura	Up to 60 minutes duration, usually 20 minutes, often visual	None	None
Associated Symptoms	Nausea, vomiting, diarrhea, conjunctival injection, stuffed nose, phonophobia, photophobia, increased sensitivity, occasional ptosis	Ipsilateral ptosis, miosis, conjunctival injection, lacrimation, stuffed and running nostril	Episodic type: loss of appetite, either photophobia or phonophobia Chronic type: photophobia or phonophobia or presence of nausea
Behavior	Retreat to a dark quiet room (hibernation)	Frenetic pacing, rocking	Generally not affected, may have mild reduction in functional capacity

The head and neck should be palpated for signs of pericranial tenderness and excessive tightening of muscles. Careful examination may demonstrate points of exquisite tenderness with or without referral of pain. These trigger points may be found in the musculature of the head and neck as well as in the sternocleidomastoid, suprascapular, and infrascapular muscles. Attention should be paid to the occiput; check for tenderness in the areas of the greater and lesser occipital nerves.

Patients may deny tightness of their neck muscles while the examination reveals excessive tightness and even spasm. Check for range of motion of the neck in all directions, adding flexion and extension to extreme turns to either side. Inquire as to whether there is any pain during these movements. Inability to flex the neck with stiffness and pain in the presence of fever may be a sign of meningitis or hemorrhage.

Apply gentle pressure to the orbits to check for orbital tenderness or increased intraocular pressure associated with glaucoma. The temporomandibular joints should be palpated for tenderness and auscultated as well. Deviation of the jaw on opening,

noise in the joint, tenderness on palpation, restricted range of motion, pain on opening wide or clenching, and spasm of the internal pterygoid muscles may be evidence of temporomandibular joint dysfunction. Examine the temporal arteries for prominence and palpate them for adequate pulsation, tenderness, or rigidity to rule out arteritis, particularly in older females.

Palpation of the frontal and maxillary sinuses may reveal tenderness and swelling, which, in the presence of stuffed nostrils, nose and sinus pain, and fever, may indicate sinusitis. You might use a pen light or an otoscope to transilluminate the frontal and maxillary sinuses in search of cloudiness. Acute sinusitis is generally associated with fever and a purulent nasal discharge. Chronic sinusitis is rarely a cause of chronic headache, although it is important to be alert to sphenoid sinusitis as a cause of chronic headache. This unusual occurrence is difficult to diagnose and may require computed tomographic imaging of the sinuses or endoscopy by an experienced otolaryngologist.

The extracranial carotid arterial tree should be palpated and auscultated, includ-

The New England Center for Headache
778 Long Ridge Road • Stamford, CT 06902 • (203) 968-1799

Neurological Examination

NAME: _____   DATE: _____

VITAL SIGNS: Thyroid _____ Handedness R _____ L _____ A _____

BP: (r) _____ (l) _____ P _____ R _____ Ht _____ Wt _____

GENERAL: _____

VASCULAR: Heart: _____

Bruits: Head _____ Eyes _____ Neck _____

Pulses: Superficial Temporal _____ Carotid _____ Others _____

HEAD: Shape _____ Size _____ Bumps _____ Tenderness _____ Greater Occipital Nerves: R _____ L _____

NECK: ROM _____ Pain _____ { Cervical Spine _____   Tenderness _____ { Cervical Spine _____
                                         { Muscles _____   { Muscles _____

MENTAL STATUS: Alert _____ Speech _____ Orientation _____ Memory { Immediate _____
                                                                                { 3' _____ Naming _____ Sentence _____

Spelling _____ Calculation _____   { 10' _____ 6 digits: Forward _____
                                                                            Backward _____

CRANIAL NERVES: ¹Smell: R _____ L _____ ²Acuity: R _____ L _____ ²Fundi: R _____ L _____ ²Visual Fields _____

³,⁴,⁶EOM _____ Convergence _____ Pupils: R _____ L _____ Response _____

Ptosis _____ Nystagmus _____ ⁵Motor _____ TMJ Pain: Opening _____ Closing _____ Palpation _____

⁵Sensory _____ Corneal Reflex: R _____ L _____ ⁷Power _____ ⁷Taste _____

⁸Hearing: R _____ L _____ Weber _____ Rinne _____ ⁹Sensory _____

⁹,¹⁰Gag/Swallow: R _____ L _____ ¹⁰Palate _____ ¹¹_____ ¹²Tongue _____

MOTOR:
0–5 R/L   Power: Arms: Proximal _____ Distal _____ Tremor _____

Legs: Proximal _____ Distal _____

Tone _____ Atrophy _____

Cerebellar   F → N: R _____ L _____ H → S: R _____ L _____

Tandem _____ Heel Walk _____ Toe Walk _____ Romberg _____

Hopping _____ Rapid Alternating Movements _____ Gait _____

SENSORY: Light Touch _____ Pin _____ Cold _____ Vibration _____

2 Pt. Discrimination _____ Stereognosis _____ DSS _____ JPS _____

REFLEX: Snout _____ Jaw Jerk _____ Palmo-mental _____ Hoffman _____

Biceps: R _____ L _____ Brachioradialis: R _____ L _____

Triceps: R _____ L _____ Knee Jerk: R _____ L _____ Ankle Jerk: R _____ L _____

Babinski: R _____ L _____

Abdominal _____

Other _____

OTHER:

Figure 5–4

Form used to record findings from the neurological examination.

ing the external carotid and vertebral arteries. Auscultation of the orbits with the stethoscope bell is also important. The presence of bruits suggests vessel disease, arteriovenous malformation, or vascular tumor, and appropriate follow-up in the form of arterial studies should be considered. We also auscultate over the temporal bone, under the angle of the jaw for the carotid artery, and at the base of the neck for the vertebral and subclavian arteries.

Palpate the neck further for signs of thyroid nodules or symmetrical or asymmetrical enlargement; look for adenopathy, which suggests an infection such as sinusitis or other diseases such as malignancy.

THE CRANIAL NERVES

An examination of the cranial nerves is essential in ruling out organic pathology. Check the patient's sense of smell in each nostril. Funduscopic examination reveals the presence or absence of papilledema or retinal changes secondary to hypertension and diabetes. Papilledema is a sign of increased intracranial pressure that may be secondary to a structural lesion or to benign idiopathic intracranial hypertension (pseudotumor cerebri).

Some studies have demonstrated that occasional cases of pseudotumor are not associated with papilledema. If the index of suspicion is high, a lumbar puncture is indicated to rule out elevated cerebral spinal fluid pressure. This might be especially important in overweight adolescent girls with irregular menses and blurred vision who have chronic daily headache that has been totally refractory to the usual treatments. Other causes include high doses of vitamin A and tetracycline, hyperparathyroidism, and Cushing's disease.

Check for visual field defects using finger counting with double simultaneous stimulation (putting fingers in both fields at once while the patient fixates on your nose). Check for diplopia as may be seen in structural pathology, demyelinating disease, and meningitis by having the patient follow your flashlight in all directions of gaze. All three sensory divisions of the fifth, or trigeminal, nerve on each side should be examined. The first division is examined by testing the corneal reflex and using touch and pin on the forehead. The second and third divisions are tested by checking light touch and pin prick on the cheek and jaw. Check the voluntary movements of muscles supplied by the motor division of the fifth cranial nerve by feeling the masseter bulk on clenching.

Pathology involving the seventh, or facial, nerve may show up as a typical Bell's palsy (paralysis of one entire side of the face). Central lesions involving the face allow patients to smile spontaneously, which is not true of peripheral lesions of the seventh nerve. The weakness from a central lesion affects only the lower two-thirds of the face and usually spares the frontalis muscle.

We test the eighth nerve by checking hearing with light finger rubbing, with a tuning fork, and by checking both the Weber and Rinne responses.

Neuralgia of the ninth, or glossopharyngeal, nerve may cause pain in the tonsillar area with radiation to the ear. The function of the ninth nerve is tested by determining whether sensation of light touch to the back of the throat is intact on each side.

The tenth nerve may affect the character of the voice and may also affect swallowing. When intact, it causes the palate to elevate symmetrically when the gag reflex is tested.

When the eleventh, or spinal accessory, nerve is impaired, a weak trapezius or sternocleidomastoid muscle may result. Shoulder shrugging and lateral head turning are weak.

Deviation of the tongue (which points to the side of the lesion) or atrophy or fasciculations of the tongue suggest lesions of the twelfth, or hypoglossal, nerve.

SENSORY SYSTEMS

Migraineurs' sensory systems are usually normal on testing.

All modalities, including light touch, pinprick, cold, and vibratory sensations, should be evaluated. Check right versus left and proximal versus distal. Many patients with migraine characteristically demonstrate coolness of the extremities which is probably due to excessive vasomotor tone in the extremities that results in decreased blood flow and decreased perception of cold stimuli distally.

During a migraine attack, patients typically report a hot head and cold hands. In fact, they find partial relief by touching their ice-cold hands to warmer areas of the head. Historically, this phenomenon has been interpreted as increased blood flow to the extracranial vasculature, resulting in enhanced heat, and similarly, decreased blood flow to the extremities, resulting in coolness.

THE MOTOR SYSTEM

Check all muscle groups for tone and strength. We spot-check proximal and distal power in the arms and legs. Look for the presence of tremor at rest or intention tremor on action. Tremors may be associated with a benign familial disorder, but they may also be signs of Parkinson's disease, medication side effects, demyelinating disease, hyperthyroidism, and anxiety. Look for cogwheel rigidity (stiffness), which suggests Parkinson's disease.

CEREBELLAR EXAMINATION

This is best accomplished by evaluating the patient's gait and checking the patient's coordination. The usual finger to nose and heel to shin test, tandem walking, and Romberg's test should be performed. Simple observation of the patient without formal testing can yield a very accurate impression of cerebellar integrity.

REFLEXES

Check all deep tendon reflexes (biceps, brachioradialis, triceps, quadriceps, Achilles) as well as pupillary and corneal reflexes. Pathological reflexes, including the plantar responses and snout and jaw jerk, should be evaluated as well. If meningitis is suspected, check for Kernig's or Brudzinski's sign, or just plain stiffness of the neck.

MENTAL STATUS

Look for signs of depression or anxiety. The history should be helpful in revealing these syndromes. Direct observation of the patient's emotional tone may reveal blunted, sad, or labile affects. Brief cognitive evaluations should be conducted. Check recent and remote memory and concentration and observe for cognitive styles that may be ruminative or obsessional. This assessment is especially important in patients who present with post-traumatic headache that is often accompanied by post–head trauma syndrome and symptoms of personality change, memory deficits, and difficulties with concentration and attention.

GENERAL PHYSICAL EXAMINATION

A general physical examination should be performed. This is important in ruling out comorbid difficulties or factors that may contribute to headache, such as hypertension, thyroid dysfunction, cardiovascular disease, asthma, or gastrointestinal disturbances.

Patients may also be taking medications associated with systemic effects. Specifically, β-blockers may produce bradycardia or wheezing; overuse of ergotamines may cause decreased peripheral pulsations, myalgia, stomach pain, and nausea. Overuse of narcotics and butalbital products may result in cerebellar ataxia, impaired concentration, sedation, and depression. Patients in withdrawal from benzodiazepines or barbiturates may exhibit symptoms of increased irritability, tremors, hyperreflexia, dilated pupils, and piloerection, and those who take narcotics on a frequent basis may exhibit miosis and sedation during acute intoxication.

Diagnosis

Diagnostic formulations can be made after a careful review of the entire medical history. When you review the IHS criteria for each of the primary headache disorders it will become obvious that the information required for making a diagnosis has been included in the history-taking format we have described. The history (with the IHS criteria) also enables you to differentiate among the various headache types. When patients have more than one type of headache, the picture is almost always one of coexistent migraine and tension-type headache. Chapter 4 examines the issues surrounding whether these headaches exist as separate entities or as a continuum. A review of the summary face sheet demonstrates that pain may start as dull or moderate and move up the scale to incapacitating, with demonstrable, clear-cut symptoms of migraine.

Although some physicians subscribe to the coexistent development of migraine and chronic tension-type headache, we prefer the concept of chronic daily headache. Chronic daily headache presents as daily dull-to-moderate pain with superimposed episodes of clear-cut, severe pain typical of migrainous events. The vast majority of patients with chronic daily headache eventually overuse analgesics or ergotamines and also have increased headache associated with drug overuse.

Thus, some authorities suggest making *chronic daily headache* a separate diagnostic category in the IHS classification schema. The majority of patients with chronic daily headache give a history of intermittent episodes of migraine that began in adolescence or during their 20s and which evolved into a pattern of chronic daily headache by their 30s or 40s. As previously described, our method of history taking and review demonstrates this phenomenon quite clearly.

Summary

Taken together, history and physical and neurological examinations provide sufficient information for making a differential diagnosis and an informed decision as to whether additional work-up is necessary. The sharing of this data with patients and their families as well as patient education and follow-up will be discussed in detail in Chapter 7.

We cannot overemphasize the importance of *patient education* in the treatment of any disorder and particularly in primary headache disorders in which there are no hard biological markers or findings on examination to substantiate patient complaints.

SUGGESTED READINGS

Bille BS: Migraine in school children. *Acta Paediatr Scand.* 1962;51(Suppl 36):1.

Blau JN: Headache history: Its importance and idiosyncrasies. *Headache Quarterly.* 1990;1(2):129.

DeJong R: *The Neurologic Examination*, 4th ed. Hagerstown, MD: Harper & Row Publishers. 1979.

Lipton RB, Silberstein SD, Stewart WF: An update on the epidemiology of migraine. *Headache.* 1994;34:319.

Roter DL, Hall JA: *Doctors Talking with Patients/Patients Talking with Doctors.* Westport, CT: Auburn Health. 1992.

Sheftell FD: Approach to the patient with headache. In Samuels MA, Feske S, Mesulam MM, et al, eds, *Office Practice of Neurology.* New York: Churchill Livingstone. (In press.)

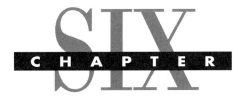

Pharmacological Treatment of Headache

Most patients are treated both by nonpharmacological methods and with medications at the time of their first visit to The New England Center for Headache. All patients begin a behavioral wellness program that includes instruction in keeping a headache calendar on which all headaches and medication use are recorded and special instructions on sleep, how and when to eat, how and why to exercise, how to relax, and how to avoid headaches by identifying possible triggers.

Although some patients receive no preventive medications, most will require medication for acute treatment of a moderate or severe headache, and, when appropriate, they receive prescriptions for preventive medications as well. We believe in using the fewest, mildest medications for the shortest amount of time possible. Some of our patients, however, do require several preventive medications.

In an effort to help our patients avoid side effects and rebound headache, we allow sufficient time during the discussion of the treatment plan to educate our patients as to how much medication is too much.

Acute Versus Preventive Therapy

The purpose of acute treatment is to prevent escalation of the attack and hopefully to reverse a moderate to severe headache and its associated symptoms. The goal of such pharmacotherapy is to restore patients to their normal functioning. Treatment may include simple or combination analgesics, butalbital-containing compounds, isometheptene-containing compounds (Midrin), antiemetics, sedatives, steroids, ergotamine tartrate, dihydroergotamine, or sumatriptan; opiates are prescribed as back-up medication in special situations.

Patients who have 3 or more days of headache-related disability per month or those who do not readily respond to any type of acute treatment receive preventive (prophylactic) medications in an effort to decrease the frequency, severity, and duration of severe headaches. Patients will continue to need acute treatment for breakthrough headaches.

General Principles of Medication Use

Analgesic rebound headache and ergotamine rebound headache are often seen in tertiary care centers. Many of our patients present with severe and frequent headaches. In a desperate attempt to keep themselves functioning and in less pain, these patients are likely to have overused medication designed for acute treatment of headache. Rather than easing their headache pain, however, such overuse usually worsens the headache syndrome and may result in dependence on medications such as opiates, barbiturates, and benzodiazepines as well as off-the-shelf analgesics. Patients are usually taken off more medications than they are given during their first visit to our Center.

REBOUND HEADACHE

The most significant causative factor in the production of intractable headaches is overuse of off-the-shelf medications, ergotamine tartrate, butalbital-containing medications, opiates, and benzodiazepines. The great majority of patients who are involved in this overuse syndrome eventually feel better after discontinuing medications. Their symptoms may worsen for a period of days or weeks, but improvement follows this initial washout period. The analgesic washout period may continue for as long as 2 to 3 months, and total recovery may not occur until washout is complete. About 20% of patients do not improve after withdrawal of offending medications, and most patients who overuse medications do not respond to typically effective preventive medications or to behavioral therapies until these pharmacological agents have been withdrawn. Overuse syndrome is a frequent and serious problem among severe headache sufferers because most physicians and patients are unaware of it and do not, as a result, look for it.

Although there is no consensus among headache specialists as to which medications are most likely to produce the rebound syndrome, most agree that aspirin, acetaminophen, butalbital-containing medications, ergots, benzodiazepines, and opiates do. It is not clear whether nonsteroidal anti-inflammatory drugs (NSAIDs), dihydroergotamine, and sumatriptan produce this syndrome.

Some authorities believe that aspirin and acetaminophen may produce rebound syndromes in doses as low as two tablets daily, and certainly at the level of four to six tablets per day. Saper (1987, 1990) has shown that ergotamine tartrate can produce rebound syndromes in doses as low as 0.5 mg twice per week. Most ergot rebounders, however, take small amounts of the drug three or four times per week or more frequently when they first notice increased headache frequency.

Treatment protocols for the rebound syndromes are straightforward but may be difficult for patients to follow. Off-the-shelf analgesics may be stopped abruptly; prescription medications should be stopped more gradually. Butalbital-containing medications and opiates should be stopped slowly and cautiously; patients taking them may require admission to a specialized, inpatient headache unit. Patients usually become much worse when an offending medication reaches a critically low dose or is discontinued. The headaches increase in intensity, become intolerable, and patients become nauseated, vomit, have difficulty sleeping, and function poorly.

Patients may be given tapering doses of Midrin or NSAIDs (eg, one tablet or capsule tid $\times$ 5 days, bid $\times$ 5 days, qd $\times$ 5 days, and then off) to help them through this difficult period, which may last as long as 2 weeks. Steroids or sedatives may also be helpful. The most effective treatment is repetitive intravenous dihydroergotamine (D.H.E. 45) given in an inpatient setting on a specialty headache unit.

Patients should be advised to avoid prn medications for mild to moderate headaches as a means of preventing recurrence of rebound headache. Education and reassurance is essential. In addition, appropriate abortive medications for moderate to severe headaches should be provided, and patients should be given specific limits as well as nonrefillable prescriptions.

SIDE EFFECTS

All medications may cause side effects, and patients must be informed of those that occur most frequently. In addition, patients should be reassured that some side effects are transitory and warned of those that necessitate telephoning their physicians. We hand out medication sheets that detail beneficial effects, adverse side effects, and warning signs that should trigger a call for medical attention. Because our goal is to avoid adverse effects whenever possible, we start patients on low doses of both acute and preventive medication and increase dosage gradually. This technique also enhances patient compliance.

PREGNANCY

Many women with migraine are of childbearing age. We warn these women not to become pregnant while taking headache medication. Preventive medication should be discontinued well in advance of attempting to become pregnant.

We permit patients who take acute migraine medication and are trying to become pregnant to take their medication from the start of their menses until the tenth day of the monthly cycle. Although it is our philosophy to withhold all medication, including off-the-shelf products, throughout the entire pregnancy, we realize that some women require treatment at times.

We make every effort to engage in a detailed discussion about medication with patients and their husbands or partners prior to the pregnancy. We also encourage open discussion between patients and their obstetricians and pediatricians. Some medications are permissible during pregnancy if absolutely necessary, but it is a matter of philosophy as to which ones, if any, should be prescribed.

PREVENTIVE MEDICATIONS

Patients should be taught that since preventive medications need 2 to 6 weeks to take effect, they should not become impatient when they perceive no immediate effect. β-Blockers and calcium channel blockers take 2 to 4 weeks to work; antidepressant medications can take as long as 3 to 6 weeks

to achieve clinical effect. Fluoxetine (Prozac) typically takes as long as 4 to 6 weeks before the onset of clinical effectiveness. We ask patients not to discontinue medications or change dosages on their own, but rather to call us for specific instructions.

Abruptly discontinuing β-blockers, antidepressants, and vasoactive medications can worsen headaches and cause other undesirable effects. We educate our patients to take responsibility for their medications, not to let the supply run out, and to keep their prescriptions current.

PROPER TIMING OF ACUTE TREATMENT

If patients treat an acute migraine very early in the attack, mild medications such as off-the-shelf analgesics may provide adequate relief. Even the most potent medications may be ineffective, however, if patients wait too long before initiating treatment.

We instruct patients not to treat mild headaches with medication but rather to use behavioral techniques as described in Chapter 7. When a headache is becoming moderately severe, patients are instructed to medicate with Midrin, NSAIDs, or Fioricet; if it is about to become incapacitating, they can switch to Imitrex, D.H.E. 45, or Cafergot. If these are not effective, we prescribe a backup medication such as Stadol NS or dexamethasone. We also provide cards that suggest to emergency room physicians what we would do if all these measures fail, and we instruct our patients to go to the local emergency room, if necessary, and show the cards.

Emergency room physicians in our area are familiar with our cards and our protocols. We recommend that any physician who routinely treats headache and is likely to send patients to emergency rooms when not on call make every effort to discuss his or her treatment plan with local emergency room physicians.

Acute Therapy for Headache

In the United States, patients prefer oral medication to suppositories. However, tablets are not as well absorbed during an acute migraine process, and some patients with nausea or vomiting are unable to take them. Suppositories should be considered in such a situation. Recently, preparations such as nasal sprays and self-administered injections have become more popular. Sublingual headache preparations became difficult to find because they were discontinued by their manufacturers, but they are now available again. Medihalers were removed from the market and are thus no longer available in the United States.

SIMPLE ANALGESICS

If taken sufficiently early and in proper doses, simple analgesics may stop the progression of an acute migraine attack or tension-type headache. Two regular aspirin tablets (650 mg) or two extra-strength acetaminophen tablets (1000 mg) may be helpful in certain patients (Table 6–1). Acetaminophen is preferred over aspirin for children and for patients with upper gastrointestinal problems; it can cause liver dysfunction if overused.

COMBINATION ANALGESICS

Caffeine acts as an adjuvant to analgesics and improves absorption from the stomach. Some patients actually treat themselves with coffee or colas that contain caffeine. Many off-the-shelf combination analgesics contain caffeine. Extra-strength Excedrin has 250 mg of aspirin, 250 mg of acetaminophen, and 65 mg of caffeine; Anacin has 400 mg of aspirin and 32 mg of caffeine. Other combination preparations contain buffering compounds and vasoactive medication, and all can be helpful in proper dosages. We permit our patients to take a maximum of two to four simple or combination analgesics up to 3 days per week, but not on a daily basis for both tension-type headache and migraine. It is important to explain to patients that 300 mg of caffeine daily (three to four cups of coffee) may be enough to produce caffeine rebound and withdrawal headaches. Some patients do poorly on even

Table 6–1

COMPOSITION OF SIMPLE OFF-THE-SHELF ANALGESICS

	Ingredients (mg)		
	Aspirin	**Acetaminophen**	**Other**
Advil			Ibuprofen 200
Aleve			Naproxen sodium 220
Anacin III		325	
Anacin III (maximum strength)		500	
Aspirin	325		
Bayer Aspirin	325		
Bayer Aspirin (8-hr time release)	625		
Bayer Aspirin (maximum)	500		
Bayer Aspirin (therapy)	325		
Datril E.S.		500	
Ecotrin (enteric-coated)	325		
Ecotrin maximum strength (enteric-coated)	500		
Empirin	325		
Ibuprofen			Ibuprofen 200
Mediprin			Ibuprofen 200
Motrin IB			Ibuprofen 200
Nuprin			Ibuprofen 200
Panadol		500	
Tylenol		325	
Tylenol (extra-strength)		500	

From Rapoport A, Sheftell F: *Conquering Headache.* Hamilton, Ontario: Empowering Press. 1995.

lower amounts. Patients must learn to add the amount of caffeine in beverages to that in medications to determine daily caffeine intake (Table 6–2).

ISOMETHEPTENE-CONTAINING MEDICATION (MIDRIN)

An effective combination analgesic containing isometheptene mucate 65 mg, acetaminophen 325 mg, and dichloralphenazone 100 mg is useful in children and adults for acute tension-type headache and migraine. Isometheptene is a sympathomimetic amine that constricts peripheral blood vessels and may work centrally. Acetaminophen is an analgesic, and dichloralphenazone is a mild tranquilizer. The usual adult dosage is two capsules stat, which may be repeated after 1 hour if needed, up to a

Table 6–2
COMPOSITION OF COMBINATION OFF-THE-SHELF ANALGESICS

	Ingredients (mg)			
	Aspirin	*Acetaminophen*	*Caffeine*	*Other*
Anacin	400		32	
Anacin (maximum strength)	500		32	
BC-Powders	650		32	Salicylamide 195
Bufferin	324			Aluminum glycinate and magnesium carbonate
Cope	421		32	Magnesium hydroxide 50 and aluminum hydroxide 50
Excedrin (extra-strength)	250	250	65	
Excedrin PM		500		Diphenhydramine citrate 38
Midol Caplet	454		32.4	Cinnamedrine HCl 14.9
Percogesic		325		Phenyltoloxamine citrate 30
Vanquish	227	194	33	Aluminum hydroxide 50 and magnesium hydroxide 50

From Rapoport A, Sheftell F: *Conquering Headache.* Hamilton, Ontario: Empowering Press. 1995.

maximum of four to five capsules per day, used up to 3 days per week; half doses are given to smaller children. Side effects are minimal and may include dizziness, drowsiness, and gastrointestinal symptoms. Contraindications include only the concomitant use of monoamine oxidase inhibitor antidepressants such as phenelzine (Nardil).

NONSTEROIDAL ANTI-INFLAMMATORY MEDICATIONS

Many of the NSAIDs are useful in treating an acute migraine attack and tension-type headache. Lack of response to one agent does not necessarily mean that others will not be helpful, so at least three NSAIDs should be tried before it is decided that this class of medication is not helpful.

Several off-the-shelf brands of ibuprofen, including Advil, Mediprin, Motrin IB, and Nuprin (200 mg per dose) are available (see Table 6–1). Naproxen sodium (Anaprox) has recently become available in a 220 mg off the-shelf tablet brand, Aleve.

We favor five types of prescription NSAIDs: naproxen sodium (Anaprox) 275 mg; meclofenamate (Meclomen) 100 mg; flurbiprofen (Ansaid) 100 mg; ketoprofen (Orudis) 75 mg; and ketorolac (Toradol) 10

mg. The dose is two tablets (one for ketorolac) or capsules stat, repeated in 1 to 4 hours if required. These medications should be taken with food and discontinued if gastrointestinal symptoms occur.

Ketorolac, the first available injectable NSAID, is given intramuscularly (30 to 60 mg) and can help relieve a migraine attack. A new sustained-release form of ketoprofen (Oruvail, 200 mg) is enteric-coated and is absorbed from the small intestine rather than from the stomach. It does not work as quickly as the short-acting form, so its best use may be when treatment is needed for several days, as in menstrual migraine.

The most frequent side effects of the NSAIDs are stomach discomfort and dyspepsia. These adverse effects can be managed with histamine blockers such as ranitidine (Zantac, 150 mg) hs or bid, or with a more specific antidote such as misoprostol (Cytotec) starting at 100 µg tid, which may cause diarrhea. The only contraindications to NSAID use are severe ulcer disease, certain types of bowel dysfunction such as Crohn's disease, clotting disorders (tendency to bleed), and concomitant use of aspirin, steroids, or alcohol. NSAIDs should be used with caution in patients who have asthma.

BUTALBITAL-CONTAINING MEDICATIONS

When off-the-shelf analgesics, Midrin, and NSAIDs have been tried and have proven ineffective, the butalbital-containing medications may provide relief. Many preparations are available; some contain codeine and all contain aspirin or acetaminophen (Table 6–3). The most frequently used are Fiorinal (aspirin 325 mg, caffeine 40 mg, and butalbital 50 mg); Fioricet and Esgic (acetaminophen 325 mg, caffeine 40 mg, and butalbital 50 mg); Phrenilin (acetaminophen 325 mg, butalbital 50 mg, without caffeine); Axotal (aspirin 650 mg, butalbital 50 mg, without caffeine); and Fiorinal with Codeine and Fioricet with Codeine, which contain 30 mg of codeine in addition to acetaminophen or aspirin, caffeine, and butalbital.

Butalbital is a short-acting barbiturate that can be very helpful in treating tension-type headache and migraine if used early in the attack but can cause rebound and dependency if used on a continuing basis. Acetaminophen-containing medications are less likely to cause adverse stomach effects. Medications that contain butalbital are so effective that patients tend to use them frequently, sometimes in advance of a severe headache to prevent its escalation. Some patients use them to treat anxiety. Patients who are very sensitive to caffeine may prefer Phrenilin or Axotal before bedtime.

The starting dose of butalbital-containing agents is one tablet or capsule stat, repeated in 1 to 2 hours up to a maximum of three per day. If this is not helpful, the medication can be given as two tablets or capsules stat, repeated in 4 to 6 hours up to a maximum of four to six per day. This dose may cause side effects. This medication should be taken no more frequently than 3 days per week; rebound headaches and dependency may occur if they are taken daily over a prolonged period.

Side effects include drowsiness, hyperactivity, ataxia, difficulty with gait, memory loss, and confusion. Patients must be cautioned not to drive or engage in any other activity that requires alertness.

OPIATES

Opiates should be used cautiously in treatment of acute migraine but can be very helpful. We prefer to start with butorphanol nasal spray (Stadol NS), a noncontrolled opioid analgesic that is readily absorbed through the nasal mucosa and is easy to use at home. Butorphanol is an agonist-antagonist that has agonist action at the kappa receptor and mixed agonist/antagonist action at the mu opiate receptor and has less abuse potential than other opioids because it does not induce euphoria while it decreases pain. Onset of activity occurs in 15 to 20 minutes with full effect within 30 to 60 minutes. Butorphanol can be used in patients who are nauseated or vomiting and can be ordered via telephone by physicians with-

Table 6–3

COMPOSITION OF THE BUTALBITAL-CONTAINING MEDICATIONS

Drug/Components	Quantity (mg)	Recommended Dosage
Fiorinal		1–2 tablets q4h as needed; no more than 6/day
Butalbital	50	
Aspirin	325	
Caffeine	40	
Fiorinal with codeine		1–2 capsules q4h as needed; no more than 4/day
Butalbital	50	
Aspirin	325	
Caffeine	40	
Codeine	30	
Fioricet		1–2 tablets q4h as needed; no more than 6/day
Butalbital	50	
Acetaminophen	325	
Caffeine	40	
Fioricet with codeine		1–2 capsules q4h as needed; no more than 4/day
Butalbital	50	
Acetaminophen	325	
Caffeine	40	
Codeine	30	
Esgic		1–2 tablets q4h as needed; no more than 6/day
Butalbital	50	
Acetaminophen	325	
Caffeine	40	
Phrenilin		1–2 tablets q4h as needed; no more than 6/day
Butalbital	50	
Acetaminophen	325	
Axotal		1–2 tablets q4h as needed; no more than 6/day
Butalbital	50	
Aspirin	650	

From Rapoport A, Sheftell F: *Conquering Headache.* Hamilton, Ontario: Empowering Press. 1995.

out triplicate prescription (in those states where it is required for scheduled opiates).

The dose is one spray in one nostril (1 mg) stat, which may be repeated in 1 hour and again 3 to 4 hours after that. Patients should be warned that they may use only one spray dose at a time, even if they do not think they received the entire dose. Butorphanol is a highly effective pain reliever and may stop the migraine process.

Side effects include sedation in a large percentage of patients; this effect may be beneficial at night or when nothing else has been effective. Patients may note dizziness, a dysphoric or drugged feeling, and confusion. Contraindications include concomitant use of other narcotics. Although some patients function well after receiving butorphanol for the first time, all should be cautioned to relax at home after their first dose. Stadol NS may be a realistic alternative to vasoconstrictors for patients with coronary artery disease and hypertension.

Other opiates including Percocet, Percodan, codeine, Darvon, Vicodin, Lortabs, Hydrocet, and DHC Plus may be helpful (Table 6–4). In special circumstances, other, stronger opiates may also be tried but should be used only occasionally, only when absolutely necessary, and only when no other medications have been helpful.

Some pain experts believe in using moderate doses of opioids on a daily basis, but we find that very few headache patients are candidates for this type of treatment. It is acceptable to give an occasional dose of intramuscular narcotics in a physician's office or emergency room. The most frequently administered drugs are meperidine (Demerol), in a dose of 75 to 100 mg, combined with promethazine (Phenergan) 50 mg, or hydroxyzine (Vistaril) 50 mg, adjuvant medications with antiemetic and/or sedative effects.

ERGOT ALKALOIDS

Ergotamine tartrate was first discovered to help headaches in the 19th century and has been available for over 50 years as Cafergot and Wigraine in tablets and suppositories. In the past it was available as a sublingual preparation, an injection, and in an inhaler. Ergotamine tartrate is erratically absorbed when taken by mouth and much better absorbed by the rectal mucosa when taken as a suppository. A Wigraine tablet contains ergotamine tartrate 1 mg and caffeine 100 mg. The Cafergot suppository contains ergotamine tartrate 2 mg and caffeine 100 mg. A sublingual preparation of ergotamine tartrate 2 mg has at times been in short supply. Starting dose of the tablet form is two tablets stat, followed by two tablets in 1 hour if required. (Cafergot tablet production has recently been discontinued. The suppositories are still available.)

When the Cafergot suppository is used, a quarter of a suppository should be taken initially and repeated in 1 hour if required. Dosage can be raised gradually if needed. Raskin (1988) suggests that a subnauseating dose be determined prior to using the medication. The maximum dose should be 4 mg per day; ergotamine should not be used more than 2 days per week. The only exception is in women with menstrually related migraine who can use ergotamine tartrate 3 days per week in the week of their menses, as long as they decrease the frequency in the other weeks of the month.

As ergotamine tartrate often exacerbates or produces nausea and vomiting, patients should be pretreated with antiemetics such as metoclopramide (Reglan) 10 mg by mouth

Table 6–4
SELECTED OPIATES AVAILABLE BY PRESCRIPTION

Opiate Name	Single-Dose Size (mg)	Recommended Dosage
Demerol (meperidine) tabs	50	1 tablet q6h; as needed ≤4/day
Dilaudid (hydromorphone) tabs	2	1 tablet q6h; as needed ≤4/day
Duragesic (transdermal system) (fentanyl)	25 μg/h	1 patch changed q72h
Levo-Dromoran (levorphanol) tabs	2	1 tablet q6h; as needed ≤4/day
MSIR tabs (morphine for immediate release)	15	1 tablet q6h; as needed ≤4/day
Stadol NS (nasal spray) (butorphanol tartrate)	1	1 spray in 1 nostril. May repeat in 1 h; then again in 4 h; as needed

From Rapoport A, Sheftell F: *Conquering Headache.* Hamilton, Ontario: Empowering Press. 1995.

or promethazine (Phenergan) 25 or 50 mg by mouth or suppository. Premedication is not necessary in patients who do not develop nausea. However, even in the absence of nausea or vomiting, metoclopramide has been shown to reduce gastric stasis, often present during migraine, and thus to enhance absorption of the oral medication to follow. Both antiemetics occasionally help the headache itself.

The major side effects of ergotamine tartrate are nausea and vomiting, abdominal pain, muscle cramps, and, rarely, distal paresthesias. Rebound headaches often occur in patients who use this medication regularly, more than 2 and certainly 3 days per week. Such overuse produces increased frequency of headaches, which respond readily to small doses of ergotamine. Before long the patient gets daily headaches and takes ergotamine daily.

Contraindications include pregnancy or plans to become pregnant, uncontrolled hypertension, coronary artery or peripheral vascular disease, sepsis, liver disease, kidney dysfunction, and concomitant use of sumatriptan. Because erythromycin, azithromycin (Zithromax) and other macrolide antibiotics decrease the metabolism of ergotamine, patients who take them should be observed for higher blood levels. Patients who take the drug in large amounts on a daily basis may develop ergotism as well as ergotamine rebound headaches. Ergotism is characterized by nausea; weakness; cold, bluish, and tingling extremities; and sometimes lack of distal pulses and arterial insufficiency.

DIHYDROERGOTAMINE (D.H.E. 45)

Dihydroergotamine is a hydrogenated form of ergotamine that has been available for 50 years in injectable form. Although it is a weaker arterial constrictor and a stronger venoconstrictor than ergotamine tartrate, it is nonetheless contraindicated in the same situations. It stimulates type 1 serotonin receptors on nerves and blood vessels and centrally in the brain stem. It has been very helpful in the treatment of acute migraine, especially in physician's offices, in emergency rooms, and in inpatient settings, and is approved for intramuscular and intravenous use in the United States. Several papers indicate that D.H.E. 45 can be effective via subcutaneous injection as well. The intranasal preparation is almost as effective as the injectable one and is available in several other countries. It may become available as Migranal in the United States in 1996.

The intramuscular or subcutaneous injection dose is usually 1 mg; it is not necessary to pretreat with an antiemetic. When given intravenously, D.H.E. 45 should be started as a 0.25 mg dose, which can be repeated after 1 hour. Used intravenously on a repetitive basis in a hospital setting, the usual test dose is 0.25 mg; the routine dose is 0.5 to 1 mg tid, given slowly over a 5-minute period by intravenous push through a heparin lock. Patients who receive the medication by this route should be pretreated 30 minutes before with an antiemetic.

The most frequently prescribed pretreatment is metoclopramide IV, 10 mg. A common side effect is akathisia, described as intense restlessness or "anxiety." We prefer to give promethazine 25 or 50 mg by mouth, or occasionally metoclopramide by mouth rather than IV.

A compounded nasal spray form of dihydroergotamine is given as 0.5 mg per spray, with a dose of one spray in each nostril. Patients repeat this in 10 minutes for a total dose of 2 mg. This regimen may be repeated in 1 hour if it has not been effective. When used intranasally, dihydroergotamine has very few side effects; those that do occur include nasal stuffiness and muscle cramps.

Although dihydroergotamine nasal spray is very effective, it may not be as effective as the injectable preparation. All forms of dihydroergotamine are safe and effective and probably work more quickly and are more effective with fewer side effects than ergotamine tartrate by mouth. D.H.E. 45 nasal spray will be a welcome addition to the group of medications for acute use in treating migraine headache.

SUMATRIPTAN (IMITREX)

Sumatriptan is a selective 5-hydroxytryptamine (5-HT, or serotonin) agonist for acute treatment of migraine. Its 1993 availability in the United States represents a major innovation in the treatment of acute migraine. Like ergotamine tartrate and D.H.E. 45, its stimulation of type 1 serotonin (inhibitory) receptors causes vasoconstriction and decreases neurogenic inflammation. Its action, however, is more selective and specific than that of either D.H.E. 45 or ergotamine tartrate. Studies do not demonstrate penetration of the blood-brain barrier, so sumatriptan appears to work at peripheral receptors, possibly in the dura (see Chapter 4). It is available as a prefilled 6 mg syringe for self-administered subcutaneous injection. Alternatively, the syringe can be loaded into a spring-activated unit for self-administration; the patient never sees a needle and uses the device by placing it against the skin of the thigh and pushing a button. It is also available as a 25 mg and a 50 mg tablet and may eventually be marketed in nasal spray and rectal suppository forms. The 6 mg preparation works quickly and often begins to relieve headache within 15 to 20 minutes, with complete relief within 30 to 60 minutes. Like D.H.E. 45, sumatriptan also reduces nausea and vomiting. It should not be given during the aura or prior to onset of pain because it does not change aura duration and does not affect pain when used prior to its onset.

The subcutaneous injection markedly reduces the severity of headache, relieves nausea, vomiting, photophobia, and phonophobia, and rapidly returns 70 to 80% of patients to a state of normal functioning. The tablets are also safe and effective but deliver less prompt relief of pain. A published study by Sheftell (1994) of 100 consecutive migraineurs treated at The New England Center for Headache showed that 84% of patients obtained effective relief from the injection in an average time of 41 minutes. This paper and others in the literature report that headache recurs in one third to one half of subjects within 24 hours and that this recurrence is usually relieved by a second dose of sumatriptan.

In terms of clinical practice, if the first dose is effective but the headache recurs within 24 hours, patients may take a second dose if their headaches are moderate to severe. For most patients, if the initial dose does not relieve pain, the second dose is not likely to provide additional benefit. The maximum dose we permit is two 6 mg injections or 300 mg in tablet form in 24 hours. We prefer that patients take this medication no more than every 3 days except under special circumstances..

Although many patients develop side effects from sumatriptan, these effects are usually not serious. Their duration is from 5 to 30 minutes, and patients rarely discontinue the medication because of side effects. The most common side effects are pain at the injection site, distal paresthesias or tingling, a warm feeling all over, heaviness, and a sensation of pressure.

If heaviness or pressure occurs in the chest or neck, it is important to rule out coronary artery spasm. The drug is contraindicated in Prinzmetal's angina, coronary artery disease, basilar and hemiplegic migraine, and uncontrolled hypertension. We recommend that patients with risk factors for coronary disease, such as a family history of coronary artery disease, high cholesterol level, hypertension, obesity, postmenopausal state, smoking habit, and lack of regular exercise be given sumatriptan only after careful consideration.

A history of asthma and multiple drug allergies may increase the risk of anaphylaxis. We recommend that all patients over the age of 40 be given their first dose of sumatriptan in a physician's office or emergency room. If heaviness of the chest occurs, they should undergo a cardiogram to rule out coronary artery spasm. Sumatriptan should be used cautiously in patients who take monoamine oxidase inhibitors (MAOIs), since serotonin is metabolized by monoamine oxidase. Sumatriptan should not be given to patients within 24 hours of their being given ergotamine tartrate or D.H.E. 45.

CORTICOSTEROIDS

We use corticosteroids as back-up medication if all of the treatments described have failed. Our usual dose is oral dexamethasone 4 to 6 mg stat with a 4 mg repeat dose in 3 hours if necessary. Dexamethasone probably works by decreasing perivascular neurogenic inflammation in the dura (see-Chap. 4). We permit our patients to take dexamethasone only one to two times per month. Occasionally, we use a 3- to 5-day pulse of steroids. Side effects are brief and occur infrequently; they include reddening of the face, slight elevation of blood pressure, gastrointestinal symptoms, and insomnia. Long-term use should be strictly avoided, as it can produce avascular bone necrosis, osteoporosis, diabetes, cataracts, hypertension, and many other serious effects. We prescribe steroids for up to 3 weeks in severe cases of cluster headache (see discussion under "Our Approach to Pharmacological Treatment").

ANTIEMETICS

Pretreatment with antiemetics should be done prior to the administration of ergotamine tartrate and in any patient who usually develops nausea with headache. Antiemetics can also be given after nausea develops. We prefer promethazine (Phenergan), metoclopramide (Reglan), or prochlorperazine (Compazine). The prokinetic drug metoclopramide tends not to cause drowsiness and is appropriate for use at work and during the day. Our usual dose is 10 mg by mouth. Promethazine 25 or 50 mg by mouth, suppository, or injection does cause drowsiness, which can be helpful when patients want to sleep. Prochlorperazine is given in a dose of 10 mg by mouth or intramuscularly, or 12.5 to 25 mg as a rectal suppository, and can be tried as a 10 mg IV dose given slowly in the emergency room. IV prochlorperazine frequently produces a dramatic improvement in the headache and alleviates nausea (Table 6–5).

Trimethobenzamide (Tigan), 200 mg suppository or 250 mg capsule, and chlorpromazine (Thorazine), 25 or 50 mg tablet or 50 or 100 mg suppository, have been helpful in some patients. We also use hydroxyzine (Vistaril), a histamine (H_1) receptor antagonist, which is a good antiemetic, pain reliever, and sedative. The usual dose is a 50

Table 6–5
ORAL ANTIEMETICS

Drug Brand Name	Generic Name	Dose
Compazine	Prochlorperazine	5- or 10-mg tablet
Emetrol	Carbohydrate Solution	1 or 2 tbsp
Phenergan	Promethazine	25- or 50-mg tablet
Reglan	Metoclopramide	10-mg tablet
Thorazine	Chlorpromazine	25- or 50-mg tablet
Tigan	Trimethobenzamide	250-mg capsule
Torecan	Thiethylperazine	10-mg tablet
Vistaril	Hydroxyzine	50-mg capsule
Zofran	Ondansetron	4-mg tablet

From Rapoport A, Sheftell F: *Conquering Headache.* Hamilton, Ontario: Empowering Press. 1995.

mg capsule, which may be repeated in 2 hours. The side effect of all these medications is drowsiness and dry mouth. Thorazine can lower blood pressure and cause dizziness. The most recently introduced antiemetic is ondansetron (Zofran), 4 mg tablet or 8 mg by IV push. Indicated for nausea secondary to chemotherapy, it is helpful in stopping intractable nausea and vomiting associated with migraine.

Preventive (Prophylactic) Migraine Treatment

All preventive medication should be started at a low dose and gradually increased over a period of several weeks to achieve a therapeutic dose. Some patients respond to very low doses. Patients must be told that a minimum of 3 to 4 weeks on a reasonable dose is necessary before a medication should be discontinued and another one tried. One preventive agent at a time is preferable, but some patients need two or even three medications, depending on the severity and frequency of their migraine (Table 6–6).

β-ADRENERGIC BLOCKING DRUGS

Although other categories of medications with fewer side effects are becoming more popular, β-blockers are the most commonly used group of preventive medications for migraine. Propranolol (Inderal) was the first

Table 6-6

SELECTED PREVENTIVE MEDICATIONS FOR TREATMENT OF MIGRAINE

Category	Generic Name	Brand Name	Category†	Generic Name	Brand Name
β-Blockers	Propranolol	Inderal	Benzodiazepines/	Lorazepam	Ativan
	Nadolol	Corgard	Major and Minor	Alprazolam	Xanax
	Metoprolol	Lopressor	Tranquilizers	Clorazepate	Tranxene
	Atenolol	Tenormin		Diazepam	Valium
	Timolol	Blocadren		Buspirone	BuSpar
	Labetalol	Trandate		Chlordiazepoxide	Librium
Calcium	Verapamil	Isoptin, Calan		Clonazepam	Klonopin
Channel	Diltiazem	Cardizem		Chlorpromazine	Thorazine
Blockers	Nimodipine	Nimotop		Perphenazine	Trilafon
	Nicardipine	Cardene		Thioridazine	Mellaril
	Nifedipine	Procardia		Trifluoperazine	Stelazine
	Flunarizine	Sibelium		Thiothixene	Navane
Ergotamines	Methysergide	Sansert		Haloperidol	Haldol
	Methylergonovine	Methergine		Fluphenazine	Prolixin
	Ergonovine Maleate	Ergotrate	Muscle Relaxants/	Carisoprodol	Soma
	Dihydroergotamine	D.H.E. 45*	Inhibitors/	Methocarbamol	Robaxin
	Phenobarb/Belladonna	Bellergal	GABA-ergics	Cyclobenzaprine	Flexeril
	Bromocriptine	Parlodel		Baclofen	Lioresal
Serotonin₂	Methysergide	Sansert		Clonazepam	Klonopin
Blockers	Cyproheptadine	Periactin	Antihistamines	Cyproheptadine	Periactin
Anticonvulsants	Divalproex Sodium	Depakote		Terfenadine	Seldane
	Diphenylhydantoin	Dilantin		Astemizole	Hismanal
	Carbamazepine	Tegretol		Loratadine	Claritin
	Primidone	Mysoline	Diuretics	Acetazolamide	Diamox
	Phenobarbital	Luminal	Steroids	Prednisone	Deltasone
	Clonazepam	Klonopin		Triamcinolone	Aristocort
Ace-Inhibitors	Enalapril	Vasotec		Dexamethasone	Decadron
	Captopril	Capoten		Beclomethasone	Vancenase, Beconase, nasal
α₂-Adrenergic	Clonidine	Catapres, Tablet or Patch		Fluticasone	Flonase, nasal
Agonists	Doxazosin Mesylate	Cardura			
Stimulants/	Lithium Carbonate	Eskalith, Lithobid			
Anti-Manics	Dextroamphetamine	Dexedrine			
	Methylphenidate	Ritalin			
	Pemoline	Cylert			

GABA, γ-aminobutyric acid.
*D.H.E. 45 nasal spray (Migranal) not yet available.
†Adjunctive treatments

β-blocker approved for treatment of migraine. Timolol (Blocadren) was the second. Propranolol was accidentally found to prevent migraine when a patient taking it for heart disease noticed that his long-standing migraine disappeared. The first controlled study of propranolol was completed in 1972; propranolol was found to be more effective than placebo. Lipophilic propranolol and metoprolol (Lopressor), which readily pass into the central nervous system, and hydrophilic atenolol (Tenormin) and nadolol (Corgard), which do not, are effective. Cardioselectivity has no bearing on efficacy. Many drugs in this category have been found to be effective in treating migraine: propranolol, atenolol, metoprolol, nadolol, and timolol. We prefer to use the short-acting form of each medication and to titrate it to the most effective dose. We may then switch to the sustained release or long-acting form. Because they have long half-lives, some medications such as atenolol and nadolol are given only once per day.

At The New England Center for Headache, we prefer to begin treatment with short-acting propranolol; when the proper dose is reached we may switch to Inderal LA (long-acting). Propranolol is started at a dose of 10 to 20 mg bid and gradually increased.

The usual effective dose is 80 to 160 mg daily but some patients respond to lower or higher doses. Nadolol is started at 20 mg per day and gradually raised to a range of 80 to 160 mg. Atenolol is started at 25 mg per day and gradually raised to 50 to 150 mg.

There are many possible side effects of β-blockers, but they often occur at higher doses or if the dosage is increased too rapidly. Side effects include fatigue, depression, impotence, reduced blood pressure and pulse rate, dizziness, weight gain, gastrointestinal side effects, reduced tolerance to physical activity, increased coldness in the extremities, and abnormal dreaming and nightmares.

β-Blockers are contraindicated in certain types of cardiac disorders, asthma, chronic lung disease, diabetes, hypoglycemia, bradycardia, hypotension, Raynaud's disease, peripheral vascular disease, and severe depression. They should probably not be used in hemiplegic or other forms of complicated migraine and possibly not in migraine with aura. If β-blockers must be discontinued, the dose must be tapered gradually over a period of several days to reduce the patients' risk of developing rebound tachycardia, angina, or anxiety.

ANTIDEPRESSANTS

The three major categories of antidepressants are the tricyclic and tetracyclic antidepressants, the selective serotonin reuptake inhibitors (SSRIs), and the MAOIs. These medications are frequently used for chronic tension-type headache and chronic daily headache and are especially helpful in patients with comorbid depression and sleep disorders.

The gold standard has always been amitriptyline (Elavil); clinical trials have hinted that the SSRIs could be beneficial in migraine prophylaxis (Table 6–7). For many years, amitriptyline has been helpful in treating atypical facial pain and other chronic pain syndromes.

Antidepressants down-regulate the serotonin 5-HT$_2$ receptor and increase the availability of serotonin and sometimes noradrenaline. Relief of headache often occurs

Table 6–7

SELECTED ANTIDEPRESSANTS USED IN THE TREATMENT OF HEADACHE

Category	Generic Name	Brand Name
Antidepressants	Amitriptyline	Elavil
	Doxepin	Sinequan, Adapin
	Nortriptyline	Pamelor, Aventyl
	Desipramine	Norpramin
	Trazodone	Desyrel
	Imipramine	Tofranil
	Amoxapine	Asendin
	Protriptyline	Vivactil
	Maprotiline	Ludiomil
Antidepressants: Newer Agents	Venlafaxine	Effexor
	Fluoxetine	Prozac
	Sertraline	Zoloft
	Paroxetine	Paxil
	Clomipramine	Anafranil
	Bupropion	Wellbutrin
	Nefazodone	Serzone
	Fluvoxamine	Luvox
Monoamine Oxidase Inhibitors	Phenelzine	Nardil
	Isocarboxazid	Marplan
	Tranylcypromine	Parnate
	Pargyline	Eutonyl

at doses well below those required for antidepressant effect, but improvement in symptoms may take 2 to 4 weeks, as is the case with depression.

Some antidepressants improve sleep (e.g., Paxil) and should be given 1 to 2 hours before bedtime, whereas others have the opposite effect and should be given in the morning. Fluoxetine can be so energizing for some patients that they may have difficulty falling asleep, even if they take it at 7 AM.

TRICYCLIC ANTIDEPRESSANTS

Amitriptyline, which had been the most common treatment for daily headache disorders, is now used somewhat less frequently because other medications cause fewer anticholinergic side effects. At The New England Center for Headache, we use doxepin (Sinequan) and nortriptyline (Pamelor) for patients who awaken too early in the morning and have trouble getting back to sleep; in addition, these two agents offer a more favorable side effect profile than amitriptyline.

For patients who have difficulty falling

asleep and who awaken early in the morning, trazodone (Desyrel) helps address both their sleep problems and depression. Desipramine (Norpramin) is less sedating during the day, as is nortriptyline. The least sedating, most alerting tricyclic agent is protriptyline (Vivactil), which is usually given in the morning. Imipramine (Tofranil) may also be helpful without causing drowsiness.

Tricyclic antidepressants must be taken for 2 to 4 weeks before headaches improve, but the sleep-promoting effects can occur within 1 to 2 days. Note, too, that patients may initially complain of anticholinergic effects, which "wear off" as they develop tolerance to the medication, in spite of periodic dosage increases.

Most of these medications are available in 10 mg doses. We usually begin with 10 mg 60 to 90 minutes before bedtime and raise the dose in 10 mg increments approximately every 5 nights as tolerated, to a target dose of 30 to 50 mg. Some patients eventually require 100 mg or more, especially if they are depressed, have significant sleep disorders, or have only partial responses at lower doses. Trazodone can be started at 50 mg and raised to 100 or 150 mg over 2 weeks. Several other medications in this category are available and can be tried if other medications are not helpful.

Each of these medications is associated with several similar side effects, many of which can be distressing. These effects include increased appetite; weight gain; drowsiness upon awakening, which usually improves during the day and wears off a few days after each new dosage increase; dry mouth; constipation; blurred vision; urinary retention; and sexual dysfunction. Desyrel may cause priapism in men, particularly when they receive doses in excess of 100 mg per day.

The tricyclics are contraindicated in patients with cardiac arrhythmias, narrow angle glaucoma, and urinary difficulties such as retention or hesitancy. Nortriptyline has a narrow therapeutic window for treatment of depression and headache, so blood levels should be monitored to make certain that a therapeutic concentration has been achieved if patients fail to do well. Blood level determinations for other tricyclics are not usually necessary. Fluoxetine may elevate tricyclic or carbamazepine levels dramatically when given concomitantly.

SELECTIVE SEROTONIN REUPTAKE INHIBITORS (SSRIs)

Drugs of this newest category of antidepressants are clearly helpful in many cases of chronic tension-type headache or chronic daily headache, but their role, if any, as preventive agents in pure migraine syndromes in the absence of comorbid depression has yet to be determined. SSRIs have many fewer side effects than do tricyclic antidepressants, and they are the drugs of choice in elderly patients, especially those with cardiac problems such as arrhythmias. SSRIs can also be given in the morning followed by tricyclic antidepressants at night to enhance the therapeutic benefit and decrease the likelihood of side effects. Fluoxetine is started at 10 mg at 7 AM and can be built up to 20 mg in 7 to 10 days. Good results can be achieved in most patients at these doses, but a few show optimum improvement when they take 30 or 40 mg in the morning. The higher doses are usually reserved for patients with severe depression or eating disorders. Patients are reminded to be patient because a therapeutic effect may not be evident for a period of 3 to 6 weeks.

Because fluoxetine has received adverse publicity, we find that we must carefully explain to patients our reasons for using it. Most understand its benefit when we explain that fluoxetine has fewer side effects than tricyclic antidepressants, is not sedating, and does not cause weight gain. We do explain that a small percentage of patients on this medication may note increased severity of their headaches.

The most common side effect of fluoxetine is mild agitation or nervousness, which begins immediately upon administration and is most evident immediately following each dose; this effect improves within 1 to 2 weeks of taking the drug. Insomnia may occur, especially if the drug is taken too late in the day; tremor, anorgasmia, and other sexual dysfunction have also been reported. Small doses of cyproheptadine (Periactin) may diminish these undesirable effects of serotonin stimulation. Patients should be warned to discontinue using fluoxetine use if they notice any alteration in mood or they feel strange. Fluoxetine should not be given to extremely depressed patients unless its effects are closely monitored. We warn patients that although they will most likely be made more alert by the drug and not gain weight, a small percentage of patients may become drowsy and may note weight gain.

The other two frequently used SSRIs are sertraline (Zoloft) and paroxetine (Paxil). Sertraline is a good antidepressant that often helps headache; its major side effect profile is one of increased gastrointestinal activity with cramping and gas. This is not usually sufficiently severe to prevent its use. Paroxetine has relatively mild side effects after an initial period in which nausea may occur. Use of all three drugs has been associated with sexual dysfunction.

Venlafaxine (Effexor) is a mixed serotonin and noradrenaline reuptake inhibitor whose efficacy in headache has not yet been studied.

Nefazodone (Serzone), a recently released antidepressant, inhibits 5-HT reuptake and downregulates 5-HT$_2$ receptors. Its efficacy in headache has not yet been evaluated.

MONOAMINE OXIDASE INHIBITORS (MAOIs)

When tricyclic antidepressants and SSRIs have not helped, an MAOI such as phenelzine can be tried. MAOIs work well in treating frequent or daily headache conditions that coexist with anxiety or depression and may be used for transformed migraine or chronic daily headache.

It is estimated that 80% of migraine sufferers who take MAOIs experience an improvement of at least 50%. We prescribe MAOIs cautiously because their use requires strict dietary limitation and extreme caution with respect to specific drug interactions. Patients must avoid foods that contain tyramine (such as red wine, cheese, paté, yogurt,

balsamic vinegar) and off-the-shelf and prescription pain medications and cold preparations that contain vasoconstrictors. Meperidine (Demerol) must be strictly avoided. Extremely serious hypertensive episodes or occasional hypotension, or both, may result if these restrictions are not strictly observed. Medications that must be avoided include isometheptene; phenylpropanolamine, a component of cold and off-the-shelf diet medications; pseudoephedrine hydrochloride (Sudafed); ephedrine; imipramine; and meperidine. Only very reliable patients should be placed on MAOIs and then only after being given careful instructions and with close follow-up.

Extreme caution should be exercised if tricyclics (amitriptyline or doxepin) and MAOIs are used together. Administration of tricyclics should be stopped for 2 weeks and then tricyclics and MAOIs started simultaneously. Imipramine **cannot** be used in conjunction with MAOIs.

Phenelzine, a monoamine oxidase-A inhibitor, is started at 15 mg early in the morning; the dose can be increased at 5- to 7-day intervals in 15 mg increments up to a total dose of 30 mg early in the morning and 30 mg at noon. The maximum dose is 75 mg per day. We prefer not to give this medication late in the day because it may cause insomnia. Side effects include insomnia, weight gain, and severe changes in blood pressure. The many contraindications include concomitant use of isometheptene, meperidine, other opiates, barbiturates, carbamazepine (Tegretol), cyclobenzaprine (Flexeril), tricyclic antidepressants, off-the-shelf cold medicines, and foods that contain tyramine. Other monoamine oxidase-A inhibitors are tranylcypromine (Parnate), and pargyline (Eutonyl). Monoamine oxidase-B inhibitors such as deprenyl (selegiline or Eldepryl) for use in Parkinson's disease do not carry such restrictions.

CALCIUM CHANNEL BLOCKING MEDICATIONS

Calcium channel antagonists are widely prescribed for migraine but may not be as effective as other types of medication. They are more effective for cluster headache than they are for migraine. When calcium channels close, they prevent calcium from entering the smooth muscle cells of blood vessel walls. This, in turn, may decrease arterial spasm and result in reduced frequency of migraine. There may also be a cerebral effect.

Of the many calcium channel blockers available in the United States, verapamil (Calan, Isoptin) and diltiazem (Cardizem) are the most frequently used. Isradipine (DynaCirc), nicardipine (Cardene), and others may also be effective. Nifedipine (Procardia) is occasionally helpful, but it is a potent vasodilator that may produce or worsen headaches. Flunarizine (Sibelium) is the most commonly used calcium antagonist in Europe and Canada but is not available in this country.

We often begin with verapamil 40 mg tid or, in patients who are sensitive to medication, half that dose. The dose is increased gradually over a period of 2 to 3 weeks up to an average of 80 mg tid. Most patients tolerate this dose well. The maximum recommended dose is 160 mg tid (480 mg per day), although some patients, especially those with cluster headache, may need higher doses.

If verapamil is not effective, we prescribe diltiazem 30 mg tid and gradually increase the dose to 60 mg tid; some patients have required higher doses. When patients are stabilized and doing well on a short-acting calcium blocker, we often switch their prescription to a long-acting preparation. The sustained release forms are sometimes not as helpful as the short-acting forms, perhaps because of decreased bioavailability.

The most common side effects of calcium channel blockers are constipation (more common with verapamil) and fluid retention, but other adverse effects include cardiac dysfunction, hypotension, and drowsiness. These medications are contraindicated in patients with previous myocardial infarction, and such cardiac conditions as congestive heart failure, heart block, bradycardia, and sick sinus syndrome, as well as hypotension. They should not be prescribed for men who are actively attempting to father children, as they reduce penetration of the egg by the sperm and act like male contraceptives. They should be used with caution if given concomitantly with β-blockers.

5-HYDROXYTRYPTAMINE₂ (SEROTONIN₂) ANTAGONISTS

Cyproheptadine is an antihistamine that has calcium channel–blocking and 5-HT₂–blocking properties. It is an effective antimigraine medication in children and less so in adults. Available as a 4 mg tablet and in a syrup, the starting dose is 1 to 2 mg an hour before bedtime. The dose can be raised to 12 mg per day or higher depending on side effects. Even small doses may cause sedation. Although children tolerate this drug without frequent side effects, adults may develop drowsiness, increased appetite, and weight gain. We often use this drug in patients who have difficulty sleeping at night. It is contraindicated in patients with glaucoma and prostate enlargement.

Pizotifen (Sandomigran) is similar to cyproheptadine and is available in Canada and in Europe but not in the United States.

Methysergide (Sansert) is one of the oldest preventive migraine drugs available in the United States. It is thought to work by blocking serotonin receptors, preventing neurogenic inflammation, and constricting blood vessels. The usual dose is a 2 mg tablet tid. Four tablets per day is the maximum dose, although some clinicians give higher doses to patients who are refractory to usual doses. Side effects include nausea, muscle cramps, and abdominal pain.

One serious potential side effect, which decreases the drug's first-line position, is retroperitoneal fibrosis or overgrowth of connective tissue around various organs. Although some headache specialists feel that this only occurs with high doses given for over 6 to 12 months, others maintain that it may develop as an idiosyncratic response and could occur at any time. A common practice is to stop giving the drug after 4 to 6 months of therapy to allow a 2- to 4-week "drug holiday" and to test for ureteral stenosis. Retroperitoneal fibrosis may disappear when patients discontinue use of the drug.

Methysergide is contraindicated in patients with coronary artery or peripheral vascular disease, and it should not be taken by patients who have trouble with venous inflammation or stomach ulcers. Vasoconstrictive abortive agents should be prescribed with caution if they are to be used in conjunction with Sansert.

ANTICONVULSANTS

Anticonvulsants have been used for many years as a preventive treatment for migraine, especially in children. Hering and Kuritzky (1992), Sorenson (1988), and Mathew (1995) have demonstrated the safety and effectiveness of enteric-coated divalproex sodium (Depakote) for migraine as well as for cluster headache and chronic daily headache. The Food and Drug Administration has recently approved Depakote for the preventive treatment of migraine.

We start divalproex sodium at a low dose, either 125 or 250 mg once per day, and increase dosage by 125 mg increments every 5 days to a target dose of 750 mg per day. Most patients can take divalproex every 12 hours. Although it is not clear how this medication works, it may raise γ-aminobutyric acid levels in the cerebrum to inhibit neuronal firing. A 750 mg dose usually produces a trough serum valproate level slightly below or in the lower therapeutic range of 50 to 100 μg per mL. If a patient is not doing as well as expected, we gradually raise the dose to produce a trough level of 75 to 100 μg per mL. Most patients show improvement in their headaches at a dose of 750 mg to 1500 mg per day.

In addition to doing occasional blood level checks, we do occasional complete blood counts and liver function tests. Divalproex sodium can cause liver failure in infants and should be used cautiously in older children.

Although there are many possible side effects, they do not occur frequently. However, one should be aware that side effects include weight gain, temporary hair loss, tremor, gastrointestinal problems, sedation, and cognitive changes. If side effects occur, they often disappear when the dose is reduced and gradually increased to therapeutic levels. Sodium valproate is contraindicated in pregnant patients because of the possibility of neural tube defects in the fetus, and it should not be used in patients with hepatic disease. Because sodium valproate may elevate levels of concomitantly used benzodiazepines and barbiturates, minor tranquilizers and butalbital-containing analgesics must be given with caution.

NONSTEROIDAL ANTI-INFLAMMATORY MEDICATIONS (NSAIDs)

The nonsteroidal anti-inflammatory medications, mentioned earlier as effective for acute treatment of migraine, can be given cautiously on a daily basis as preventive agents. They are often helpful in menstrual migraine when started about 4 days before menses and continued until the period of increased headache risk has passed. For headache related to the menstrual cycle, we prefer naproxen sodium 275 mg or 550 mg tid with meals (or off-the-shelf 220 mg Aleve), but many other NSAIDs are also effective (Table 6–8). NSAIDs can be given on

Table 6–8

SELECTED NONSTEROIDAL ANTI-INFLAMMATORY MEDICATIONS FOR THE PREVENTION OF MIGRAINE

Generic Name	Brand Name
Ibuprofen	Advil, Nuprin, Motrin-IB
Meclofenamate	Meclomen
Naproxen Sodium	Anaprox
Naproxen	Naprosyn
Sulindac	Clinoril
Diflunisal	Dolobid
Ketoprofen	Orudis (Oruvail-Sustained Release)
Piroxicam	Feldene
Flurbiprofen	Ansaid
Indomethacin	Indocin
Diclofenac	Voltaren
Fenoprofen	Nalfon
Ketorolac	Toradol, PO or IM
Nabumetone	Relafen
Oxaprozin	Daypro
Etodolac	Lodine

IM, intramuscularly; PO, orally.

a chronic basis as long as they do not cause significant gastrointestinal side effects such as gastric ulceration, dyspepsia, gastritis, diarrhea, and exacerbation of clotting difficulties or de novo increase in bleeding. We often prescribe liquid antacid medications (Maalox or ALternaGEL) or histamine$_2$ (H$_2$) blockers such as ranitidine (Zantac) 150 mg hs or bid to prevent upper gastrointestinal discomfort. Misoprostol (Cytotec) can also be helpful, as can sucralfate (Carafate) and omeprazole (Prilosec).

Ketoprofen is available as a sustained-release capsule, Oruvail 200 mg. Given once daily, ketoprofen bypasses the stomach and dissolves in the small intestine. Lack of absorption from the stomach should cause fewer gastric side effects. Thus far the drug has not been proven effective in headache treatment. Indomethacin-responsive headaches are discussed in Chapter 2.

ERGOTAMINE DERIVATIVES

Ergonovine (Ergotrate or Ergometrine) has been used for over 60 years to prevent migraine but is currently not commercially available. Instead, a closely related product methylergonovine (Methergine) can be taken at a dose of 0.2 mg tid. This low dose can be raised slowly to 0.4 mg tid. Side effects occur very infrequently and include cramps, hallucinations, and chest pain.

Methylergonovine has the same contraindications as other ergot alkaloids but can be taken on a daily basis rather than only once per week. It may provide relief for some migraineurs who have not responded to any of the other medications described.

α$_2$-ADRENOCEPTOR AGONISTS

Clonidine (Catapres) is an α$_2$-adrenoceptor agonist used in the treatment of migraine, especially in the perimenopausal years, and in the prevention of sympathetic withdrawal symptomatology in patients who are undergoing detoxification from opiates. It also helps nicotine users stop their use of nicotine. It may stabilize peripheral blood vessels by inhibiting the firing of neurons (due to decreased release of noradrenaline) in the locus coeruleus in the pons. The usual dose is half of a 0.1 mg tablet twice or three times per day. The dose can be raised slowly to 0.3 mg per day, but many young healthy patients with low blood pressure cannot tolerate this level.

Clonidine is also available as a Catapres skin patch in three doses of 0.1, 0.2, and 0.3 mg. Each patch is worn for 1 week and delivers a steady dose throughout the day. The most common side effects are drowsiness, dizziness, and hypotension. Clonidine should be used cautiously in conjunction with β-blockers and other antihypertensive medications.

LITHIUM

Lithium carbonate is used frequently as a preventive medication in cluster headache but on occasion can be helpful in treating migraine. Patients must avoid dehydration and excessive salt intake; serum drug levels should be monitored at frequent intervals. The average starting dose is 150 mg bid, and the maximum dose is usually 900 to 1200 mg per day. Side effects include tremor and confusion. Lithium carbonate should be used cautiously in conjunction with calcium channel blockers, Prozac and other SSRIs, and diuretics.

STIMULANT MEDICATIONS

Stimulant medications such as dextroamphetamine (Dexedrine), methylphenidate (Ritalin), and pemoline (Cylert) are not usually used for headache syndromes, but they can reduce the frequency and severity of migraine and other headaches. These modifications can be tried in patients who have not responded to any other form of treatment, especially if they have a history of attention deficit disorder. The medications work by stimulating the ascending reticular formation in the brain stem and increasing sympathetic activity. Dexedrine is started as a 5 mg tablet, Ritalin as a 5 mg tablet, and Cylert as an 18.75 mg tablet. The doses can be raised gradually. The side effects are few and tend to be those of excessive sympathetic stimulation such as tachycardia, insomnia, and anorexia with weight loss.

BENZODIAZEPINES

Benzodiazepines are not helpful as preventive medication in pure migraine syndromes. However, patients with migraine who have comorbid anxiety disorder or panic attacks may experience improvement with daily benzodiazepines. Although these drugs can be effective as relaxants, they can be addictive, difficult to control, and may worsen headache syndromes. Buspirone (BuSpar), an anti-anxiety medication that is neither a benzodiazepine nor considered addictive, can be used on a daily basis at a dose of 10 to 20 mg tid. Other helpful medications, all of which are benzodiazepines, include lorazepam (Ativan), alprazolam (Xanax), diazepam (Valium), and chlorazepate (Tranxene).

HORMONAL THERAPY

Women who have either pure menstrual migraine (attacks occurring exclusively during menses) or a marked worsening of their migraine perimenstrually, can be effectively treated with NSAIDs starting 4 days prior to menses and continuing until the end of menses. Alternatively, such women can use the 0.05 mg Estraderm skin patch (estradiol) or oral estradiol (Estrace 1 or 2 mg) on the same schedule as the NSAIDs.

Hormone-mediated (menstrual) headaches are induced by declining levels of estradiol-17β just prior to menses. Thus, shutting off prostaglandin formation with anti-inflammatory medications or producing a boost in estrogen levels can be beneficial. Other attempts at hormonal control have been made with tamoxifen (Nolvadex), an anti-estrogen compound given in a dose of 5 to 15 mg per day during the luteal phase prior to menses; and with danazol (Danocrine), an androgen given in a dose of 200 to 600 mg per day prior to and during menses. We refer patients for gynecological consultation when we want to use these medications as part of a headache treatment protocol.

OTHER AGENTS

The herb feverfew (*Tanacetum* or *Chrysanthemum parthenium*) appears to reduce the synthesis of prostaglandins and also affects platelet aggregation. Taken on a daily basis, it may reduce the frequency of migraine attacks.

Papaverine, a vasodilator, may decrease the frequency of migraine. Although a dose of 300 to 600 mg per day is usually well tolerated, its effectiveness is questionable; the major side effects of papaverine use are nausea and drowsiness.

Calcitonin is a polypeptide hormone secreted by the thyroid gland. Its exact mode of action is not known, but it is thought to increase levels of β-endorphin, adrenocorticotropic hormone, and cortisol. The usual dose is 100 U per day (injection or nasal spray) for 10 days.

Patients who have daily severe headaches that are refractory to maximal outpatient interventions or have analgesic or ergot dependency or comorbid disorders may require inpatient treatment. Repetitive IV D.H.E. 45 has been the pharmacological mainstay for this group. This will be described fully in Chapter 10.

Our Approach to Pharmacological Treatment

The following delineates our approach to pharmacological treatment when patients first present to us. This approach is described as a continuation of the clinical cases presented in Chapter 2.

To review briefly the case of *SR*, this female patient has migraine without aura; her attacks occur infrequently, and some are associated with menses. This patient can be treated in a variety of ways.

Step One: Assuming that off-the-shelf analgesics have been ineffective, we might begin with Midrin and give two capsules stat at the beginning of a headache and repeat two capsules in 1 hour if necessary. We could also use one of several nonsteroidal anti-inflammatory compounds, such as naproxen sodium, either the prescription form or the off-the-shelf Aleve. We instruct our patients to take NSAIDs with food. Another alternative would be to start with 50 mg of Phenergan or 10 mg of Reglan by mouth followed in approximately 20 minutes by two ergotamine tartrate tablets with two more in 1 hour if necessary.

Step Two. If the techniques outlined in Step One did not help, the next step could be dihydroergotamine nasal spray in a 2 mg dose. Migranal is not yet available in the United States. Alternatively, Imitrex could be given as a subcutaneous self-injection (6 mg) when rapid return to functioning is essential or if vomiting occurs early in the attack; another injection may be given after 1 hour, for a total of two within 24 hours, if the headache does not significantly improve or recurs within 24 hours. Another option would be to give a 25 mg Imitrex tablet; this dose could be repeated after 2 hours for a total oral dose of 300 mg per day.

Finally, butorphanol nasal spray (Stadol NS) can be used, especially if the patient is at home and wants to go to sleep. The dose is one spray in one nostril (1 mg), which may be repeated in 1 hour and again in 4 hours. Some patients find this very effective in relieving pain, and it often helps them get to sleep. Butorphanol is an appropriate middle-of-the-night medication and can also be used as a back-up when other migraine medications have failed to work.

The next case, that of *JS*, is an example of migraine with aura. Treatment would be similar to treatment of migraine without aura. Some headache specialists would suggest withholding strong vasoactive medications such as Cafergot, D.H.E. 45 by nasal spray or injection, and sumatriptan during the aura. Our experience is that treatment with ergotamine tartrate or D.H.E. 45 during the aura usually shortens it and is still effective in blocking the ensuing headache.

We have seen no complications with the use of these medications prior to headache onset, although they can theoretically prolong aura symptoms. Sumatriptan does not affect the aura and does not prevent the ensuing headache. Thus, sumatriptan should be given only after headache pain begins.

Both of these patients have a low frequency of migraine, and preventive medications would not be considered. We would recommend such behavioral interventions as keeping a calendar, avoiding migraine-triggering foods, starting an exercise program, and possibly instituting biofeedback training. These behavioral approaches are appropriate for most headache patients.

TENSION-TYPE HEADACHE

For *GW*, a female patient with occasional episodic tension-type headaches, treatment would start with any one of various off-the-shelf analgesics. Some patients prefer Excedrin with 65 mg of caffeine; dosage would be two tablets stat with a repeat of one or two tablets in 4 hours. Patients who prefer no aspirin could take two Extra Strength Tylenol. Two ibuprofen tablets 200 mg each or two Aleve tablets (220 mg naproxen sodium per tablet) can also be tried and may be repeated in 2 to 4 hours. If it is necessary to prescribe medication, our choices would be two Midrin stat, or one Fiorinal or Fioricet. Some patients need two of these tablets at first, but many do not. More potent yet would be Fiorinal with codeine, Fioricet with codeine, or Stadol Nasal Spray. Patients should be cautioned not to use analgesics more than 3 days per week to prevent analgesic rebound headache.

As for *SW*, who has developed almost daily tension-type headache, her headaches also increase in frequency around her menses. She is using analgesics within reasonable limits and has not developed analgesic rebound. Thus, she could use the same off-the-shelf or prescription analgesics mentioned for the previous case, but she must limit use of these medications to 3 days per week, which may be difficult because of the frequency of her headaches.

When patients need to use analgesics more than 3 days per week, we suggest that they use different categories of medication, each one no more than 3 days per week. *SW* could, for example, use a nonsteroidal anti-inflammatory medication up to 3 days per week and take Midrin or Fioricet on another 3 days per week. We believe that varying the type of analgesic used reduces the risk of developing analgesic rebound headache and also dependency and addiction.

CHRONIC DAILY HEADACHE

The next patient, *AH*, who has chronic daily headache, is also clinically depressed. *AH* overuses acetaminophen and butalbital-containing medications without significant relief. Her headaches, which are probably migraine, usually occur around her menses.

AH's treatment is more complex and involves several steps. First, all her pain medications must be gradually withdrawn. We would attempt this on an outpatient basis, but if she is unable to tolerate the pain and disability produced by withdrawal of analgesics, we would consider her a good candidate for inpatient headache therapy. We would establish a schedule of gradual withdrawal of pain tablets. Our patients usually decrease their dosage by one tablet every other day, starting from the average number they use per day. For 1 to 2 weeks we may place them on Midrin, starting with a dose of one capsule qid for 3 days and decreasing to tid for 3 days, bid for 3 days, and qd for 3 days. This may help relieve headache during the analgesic withdrawal period.

Other alternatives during the withdrawal period are Decadron, a Medrol dose pack, or decreasing doses of nonsteroidal anti-inflammatory medications. Once analgesic-dependent patients have withdrawn from analgesic medications and their headaches stabilize, a decision can be made as to what type of preventive pharmacological treatment would be most beneficial.

Our initial prescription following analgesic withdrawal is most likely to be a tricyclic antidepressant or a selective serotonin reuptake inhibitor in low doses. We would gradually increase dosage until clinically effective levels have been reached. We give patients who are sleeping poorly doxepin, nortriptyline, or trazodone 1 to 2 hours before bedtime. For patients concerned about weight gain who do not have difficulty sleeping we might try fluoxetine, sertraline, or paroxetine.

For patients who have more migrainous episodes or are difficult to control, we may add a β-blocker such as nadolol or propranolol or, alternatively, a calcium channel blocker such as verapamil or diltiazem. Divalproex sodium or methylergonovine can also be very effective in this situation.

We have not presented a case of pure menstrual migraine unassociated with other types of headache. We treat these patients with the same acute care medications we recommend or prescribe for regular migraine patients. However, we sometimes try to prevent the pain associated with the period. If a woman can accurately predict the day her menses will start and thus the approximate day the headache will start, we ask her to take naproxen sodium from 4 days before the estimated headache day until the end of menses. The dose is either 220 mg of Aleve (off-the-shelf) or 275 mg of Anaprox by prescription tid or, occasionally, double that dose. This medication is taken with meals for approximately 8 to 10 days, depending on the length of the menses. In approximately 30 to 50% of cases, women find that their migraine attacks are either prevented or are much less severe.

When this technique does not work, we sometimes boost estrogen levels during the same time frame. One such treatment would be to use the 0.05 mg Estraderm patch beginning 4 days prior to the headache and continuing until the cessation of bleeding. Alternatively, the patient can try 1 mg of Estrace per day orally or sublingually during the same time frame.

When menopausal women on hormone replacement therapy get headaches on a monthly basis, we frequently note that they take large doses of estrogen and progesterone in a cyclical manner. Gynecologists commonly prescribe replacement estrogens in the form of Premarin (conjugated estrogens) for approximately 21 days, followed by 7 days during which it is not taken. Progesterone is usually given as 10 mg of Provera for 10 days per month. We note that patients feel worse on the days they take no estrogen and worse yet on the days they do take progesterone. Thus, we suggest that these women's gynecologists substitute low doses of pure estradiol with the 0.05 mg Estraderm patch or Estrace 1 mg given continuously throughout the month. We also recommend that progesterone be given as a 2.5 mg dose, also on a daily basis. This change in tactics decreases cyclical headaches in well over 50% of patients.

CLUSTER HEADACHE

Our last case is *LK*, a male with severe cluster headache attacks. Our approach to his headaches is to initially prescribe preventive medication beginning with verapamil 80 mg tid, raising the dose to between four and six tablets spread out throughout the day. We prefer short-acting verapamil to the long-acting forms and find that many patients require higher doses. To this we might add low doses of lithium carbonate (150 mg bid), adding more as needed.

We often prescribe oral ergotamine tartrate (one tablet bid or two tablets before bedtime if most headaches occur at night) for cluster headache patients under the age of 50 with no history of coronary artery disease. Other effective forms of therapy include 3 weeks of high-dose oral steroid therapy in gradually decreasing doses starting at 60 mg prednisone per day, methysergide in a dose of 2 mg tid, methylergonovine in a dose of 0.2 mg tid or higher, and indomethacin (Indocin) 25 mg tid or higher. Divalproex sodium is sometimes beneficial at a dose of 250 to 500 mg bid. If breakthrough headaches occur, cluster patients should receive at least 7 L/minute oxygen via a mask that fits loosely over the nose and mouth; during this treatment, patients should be seated and bending forward.

Cluster patients with breakthrough headaches can also be treated with ergots in the form of Cafergot suppositories or Wigraine tablets, or sublingual ergotamine tartrate if it is available. D.H.E. 45 injections and nasal spray, when it becomes available, may be helpful.

Although sumatriptan by subcutaneous injection has not been approved for cluster headache by the FDA, it has been shown in studies in Scandinavia and Europe to be rapidly effective in many patients. The behavioral treatment for cluster patients is avoidance of alcohol and napping during the day during the cluster period.

Two experimental therapies were shown to be effective in small numbers of patients. Marks and colleagues (1993) described application of capsaicin (Zostrix cream) to the inside of the nostril on the affected side for 7 to 10 days. Lee Kudrow (personal communication) demonstrated that bright light therapy may help to stop a cluster period. This may work by changing the sleep/wake cycle, which may be accomplished by other means as well. Use of 4% lidocaine drops in the ipsilateral nostril is not usually helpful. Spraying cocaine on the sphenopalatine ganglion daily is reported effective but has been avoided by headache specialists because it may produce dependency.

SUGGESTED READINGS

Albers GW, Simon LT, Hamik A, et al: Nifedipine versus propranolol for the initial prophylaxis in migraine. *Headache.* 1989;29:215.

Anderson AR, Tfelt-Hansen P, Lassen NA: The effect of ergotamine and dihydroergotamine on cerebral blood flow in man. *Stroke.* 1987;18:120.

Anthony M, Lance JW: Monoamine oxidase inhibition in the treatment of migraine. *Arch Neurol.* 1969; 21:263.

Belgrade MJ, Ling LJ, Sahleevogt MB, et al: Comparison of single dose meperidine, butorphanol and dihydroergotamine in the treatment of vascular headache. *Neurology.* 1989;39:590.

Boofe FJ: *The Story of Ergot.* Basel: S. Karger, 1970.

Buring JE, Peto R, Hennekens CH: Low-dose aspirin for migraine prophylaxis. *JAMA.* 1990;264:1711–1713.

Cady RK, Wendt JK, Kircher JR, et al: Treatment of acute migraine with subcutaneous sumatriptan. *JAMA.* 1991;265:2831.

Callaham M, Raskin N: A controlled study of dihydroergotamine in the treatment of acute migraine headache. *Headache.* 1986;26:168–171.

Carstairs LS: Headache and gastric emptying time. *Postgrad Med J.* 1958;51:790.

Couch JR, Ziegler DK, Hassanein R: Amitriptyline in the prophylaxis of migraine. *Neurology.* 1976;26:121.

Diamond S: Treatment of migraine with isometheptene,

acetaminophen, and dichloralphenazone combination: A double-blind, crossover trial. *Headache.* 1976;15:282.

Diamond S, Baltes B: Chronic tension headache treated with amitriptyline: A double-blind study. *Headache.* 1971;11:110.

Diamond S, Freitag FG, Diamond ML, et al: Transnasal butorphanol in the treatment of migraine headache pain. *Headache Q.* 1992;3:160–167.

Diamond S, Medina JL: Double-blind study of propranolol for migraine prophylaxis. *Headache.* 1976: 16:238.

Edmeads J: Management of acute attack of migraine. *Headache.* 1973;13:91.

Foster CA, Bafaloukos J: Paroxetine in the treatment of chronic daily headache. *Headache.* 1994;34:587–589.

Friedman MD, Wilson EJ: Migraine: Its treatment with dihydroergotamine. *Ohio State Med J.* 1947;43:934.

Gallagher RM, ed: *Drug Therapy for Headache.* New York: Marcel Dekker, Inc. 1991.

Graham JR: Cardiac and pulmonary fibrosis during methysergide therapy for headache. *Am J Med Sci.* 1967;254:23.

Greenberg DA: Calcium channels and calcium channel antagonists. *Ann Neurol.* 1987;21:317.

Hakkarainen H, Allonen H: Ergotamine vs. metoclopramide vs. their combination in acute migraine attacks. *Headache.* 1984;22:10.

Hering R, Kuritzky A: Sodium valproate in the prophylactic treatment of migraine: A double-blind study versus placebo. *Cephalalgia.* 1992;12:81.

Klapper JA, Stanton JS: Ketorolac versus DHE and metoclopramide in the treatment of migraine headaches. *Headache.* 1991;31:523.

Lance JW, Currant DA: Treatment of chronic tension headache. *Lancet.* 1964;1:1236.

Lane PL, Ross R: Intravenous chlorpromazine—Preliminary results in acute migraine. *Headache.* 1958; 25:302.

Laska EM, Sunshine A, Mueller F, et al: Caffeine as an analgesic adjunct. *JAMA.* 1984;251:1711.

Marks DR, Rapoport A, Padla D, et al: A double-blind placebo-controlled trial of intranasal capsaicin for cluster headache. *Cephalalgia.* 1993;12:114.

Mathew NT, Saper JR, Silberstein SD: Migraine prophylaxis with divalproex. *Arch Neurol.* 1995;52:281.

Medina JL: Cyclical migraine: A disorder responsive to lithium carbonate. *Psychosomatics.* 1982;23:625.

Nestrold K, Kloster R, Partinen M, et al: Treatment of acute migraine attack: Naproxen and placebo compared. *Cephalalgia.* 1985;5:115.

Olerud B, Gustavsson C-L, Furberg B: Nadolol and propranolol in migraine management. *Headache.* 1986; 26:490.

The Oral Sumatriptan Dose–Defining Study Group: An oral dose defining study. *Eur Neurol.* 1991;31:301.

Peatfield RC, Petty RG, Rose FC: Double-blind comparison of mefanamic acid and acetaminophen (paracetamol) in migraine. *Cephalalgia.* 1983;3:129.

Peroutka SJ: The pharmacology of calcium channel antagonists: A novel class of anti-migraine agents. *Headache.* 1983;23:278.

Peters BH, Fraim CJ, Masel BE: Comparison of 650 mg aspirin and 1000 mg acetaminophen with each other and placebo in moderately severe headache. *Am J Med.* 1983;76:36.

Pradalier A, Clapin A, Dry J: Treatment review: Nonsteroidal anti-inflammatory drugs in the treatment and

long-term prevention of migraine attacks. *Headache.* 1988;28:550.

Rapoport AM: Severe headache: Focus on migraine. *Neurology.* 1994;44(Suppl 3):95.

Rapoport AM, Lipton RB: Pharmacological treatment of migraine. In Samuels MA, Feske S, Mesulam MM, et al, eds, *Office Practice of Neurology.* New York: Churchill Livingstone. (In press.)

Rapoport AM, Visser WH, Culter NR, et al: Oral sumatriptan in preventing headache recurrence after treatment of migraine attacks with subcutaneous sumatriptan. *Neurology.* 1995;45:1505.

Rapoport A, Weeks R, Sheftell F, et al: Analgesic rebound headache: Theoretical and practical implications. *Cephalalgia.* 1985;5(Suppl 3):448–449.

Raskin NH: *Headache,* 2nd ed. New York: Churchill Livingstone. 1988.

Ross-Lee L, Eadie MJ, Tyrer JH: Aspirin treatment of migraine attacks: Clinical observations. *Cephalalgia.* 1982;2:71.

Saadah HA: Abortive headache therapy in the office with intravenous dihydroergotamine in the treatment of acute migraine headache. *Headache.* 1992;32:143–146.

Saper JR: TCA and MAOI therapy. *Topics in Pain Management.* 1990;5:25.

Saper JR: Ergotamine dependency: A review. *Headache.* 1987;27:435.

Saper JR, Silberstein SD, Lake AE, et al: Double-blind trial of fluoxetine: Chronic daily headache and migraine. *Headache.* 1994;34:497–502.

Sheftell FD: Chronic daily headache. *Neurology.* 1992;42(Suppl 12):32.

Sheftell FD, Silberstein SD, Rapoport AM, et al: Drug treatments for chronic headache. *Drug Therapy.* 1992;22:47.

Sheftell FD, Silberstein SD, Rapoport AM: Migraine and women: Diagnosis, pathophysiology and treatment. *J Women's Health.* 1992;1:5.

Sheftell FD, Weeks RE, Rapoport AM, et al: Subcutaneous sumatriptan in a clinical setting: The first 100 consecutive patients with acute migraine in a tertiary care center. *Headache.* 1994;34:67.

Sicuteri F: Prophylactic and therapeutic properties of l-methyl-lysergic acid butanolamide in migraine. *Int Arch Allergy Appl Immunol.* 1959;15:300.

Sicuteri F, Michelacci S, Anselmi B: Characterization of the vasoactive and anti-migraine properties of indomethacin, a new anti-inflammatory agent derived from indole. *Settim Med (Italy).* 1964;52:335.

Siegel S, Rapoport AM, Sheftell FD: Management of primary headache disorders. *Contemp Inter Med.* 1993;5;11:19.

Sorenson KV: Valproate: A new drug in migraine prophylaxis. *Acta Neurol Scand.* 1988;78:346.

Welch KMA, Darnley D, Simkins RT: The role of estrogen in migraine: A review and hypothesis. *Cephalalgia.* 1984;4:227–236.

Welch KMA, Ellis DJ, Keenan PA: Successful migraine prophylaxis with naproxen sodium. *Neurology.* 1985;34:1304.

Yrill GM, Swinburn WR, Liversedge LA: A double-blind crossover trial of isometheptene mucate compound and ergotamine in migraine. *Br J Clin Pract.* 1972;26:76.

Ziegler D: The treatment of migraine. In Dalessio DJ, ed, *Wolff's Headache and Other Head Pain,* 5th ed. New York: Oxford University Press. 1987.

SEVEN

CHAPTER

Nonpharmacological
Measures and
Physician Strategies for
Improved Outcome
of Therapy

When one thinks of nonpharmacological approaches to primary headache disorders, techniques such as biofeedback, acupuncture, and physical therapy come to mind. Sometimes we use nonpharmacological approaches without being completely aware that we are doing so. For example, the physician-patient relationship; patient education; enlisting active patient participation and responsibility in treatment; and giving advice about life-style, exercise, diet, and nutrition all qualify as nonpharmacological approaches to treatment of headache.

If these key issues are not addressed, even the best "cookbook" approaches may not exert their full beneficial effects. Compliance and treatment outcomes are more likely to be positive when nonpharmacological modalities are incorporated into the management of primary headache disorders. This chapter addresses these issues, delineates behavioral medicine as it applies to primary headache disorders, reviews patient education techniques, and suggests means

by which patient participation can be encouraged and enhanced. We will also review the usual nonpharmacological approaches from the point of view of active versus passive techniques.

Physician Strategies for Improved Outcome of Therapy

THE PHYSICIAN-PATIENT RELATIONSHIP

Roter and Hall, in their book *Doctors Talking with Patients/Patients Talking with Doctors* (1992), provide a wealth of material that sheds light on various aspects of the physician-patient relationship, and we believe this book should be required reading for physicians and patients alike.

Roter and Hall review and define four basic types of physician-patient relationships based on various degrees of physician and patient control. When physician control is high and patient control low, the relationship is defined as *paternalism*, the "doctor knows best" relationship in which the physician is in the active role and the patient is the passive recipient of advice and counsel. Decision-making is relegated primarily to the physician rather than to the patient. The opposite of this relationship occurs where patient control is high and physician control is low; this is known as *consumerism*. In this case, the patient may be in the driver's seat, and the physician is cooperative and accommodating to the patient's request for information and services. When both physician and patient control are low, the relationship is characterized as *default,* where neither party exerts control; in this situation, patients are likely to drop out of care secondary to frustration.

Finally, there is a relationship characterized as *mutuality,* in which both physician and patient control are high and the patient's job is to become part of a joint venture. You might think about which particular style is best suited for most patients. We believe that **the physician-patient relationship should be an alliance or partnership characterized by mutual respect and a spirit of collaboration.** We cannot overemphasize how vital it is that patients be believed, particularly when the issue is subjective complaints such as primary headache disorders. Physician skepticism as to the validity of patients' complaints or debility is counterproductive to open communication, is likely to produce compliance problems, and ultimately undermines the physician-patient relationship. Often, noncompliance is the only way that patients can exert control over their treatment, albeit destructively. This is, in fact, passive-aggressive behavior, born of a sense of helplessness.

EDUCATION

Time spent educating patients about diagnosis, pathophysiology, and treatment alternatives is time well-spent and goes a long way in helping to maximize compliance. The belief that an educated patient is a dangerous one is the antithesis of the truth. Education about pathophysiology of primary headache disorders is especially important to patients because there are no biological markers or clear-cut, objective, demonstrable evidence. Patients who do not understand the processes underlying their headaches may fear that they are crazy or have a more serious, undiagnosed problem. After completing the history and physical examination, physicians should, in a sit-down conference, review all findings and discuss diagnostic formulations with the patient and his or her significant others. It is important not to use medical jargon; concepts should be discussed in language patients can readily understand.

In an earlier chapter (Chap. 4) we reviewed the "stick of dynamite" educational tool (Fig. 7–1). In reviewing the causes of migraine, patients should be told that they have a biologically based disorder represented by a stick of dynamite which is in all likelihood genetic and familial. Many internal and external triggers can ignite the fuse. We explain that migraine is as valid a biological disorder as ulcer, heart disease, hypertension, and asthma, adding that once that biological vulnerability is present, a variety of factors may trigger individual attacks.

For female patients, we review the role of hormones and explain that prior to puberty, the incidence of migraine is slightly greater in boys than girls but that the incidence (number of new patients developing migraine per year) begins to rise rather dramatically among women and girls who have reached menarche. Migraine is often associated with the menstrual cycle and can be exacerbated by the use of oral contraceptives or by hormone replacement therapy. Seventy-five percent of women go into remission during the final 6 months of pregnancy but may experience an increase in migraine attacks shortly following delivery. In addition, many women experience an increase in migraine attacks during the perimenopausal period.

Our discussion with patients continues as we review the role of diet and point out that of all foods, alcohol is highest on the list of

Migraine Trigger Factors

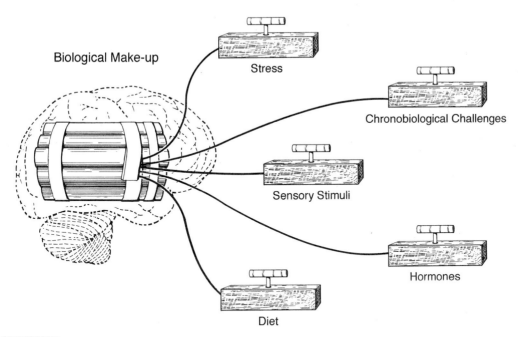

Figure 7–1

Representation of the various migraine trigger factors that can set off a headache in patients who have inherited the physiological susceptibility to migraine.

those likely to provoke attacks. We review the various other dietary provocateurs as explained in Chapter 4.

Changes such as weather, seasons, traveling through time zones, too much or too little sleep, erratic schedules, change of work shifts, and delaying or skipping meals may provoke attacks. Sensory stimuli such as strong or flickering light, heat, and odors such as perfume and cigarette smoke may also provoke attacks.

Last but not least, we explain the role of stress and psychological factors. We use diabetes as an analogy to explain to patients that even diabetic patients whose condition is well controlled with insulin may require upward adjustment of insulin when they undergo periods of marked physical or emotional duress. The same is true of any medical disorder and is no less true of migraine. We make certain that our patients understand that migraine is much more likely to occur after stressful times and during letdown periods, such as the first few days of a vacation.

Psychological factors and their relationship to primary headache disorders are discussed in Chapter 8 in great detail. Keep in mind that patients are extremely sensitive to being told that their headaches are "all in their mind" or caused by stress alone. We tell patients that if they lacked the biological vulnerability they would be less likely to get headaches, irrespective of their psychobehavioral profiles. Similarly, conditions such as irritable bowel syndrome, ulcer, hypertension, and angina are also more likely to occur in biologically vulnerable individuals.

The discussion of treatment modalities often begins with nonpharmacological approaches, which may include attempts to identify and reduce known trigger factors. For patients in whom the attack frequency of migraine is high, we explain that daily preventive medication can be used to decrease the frequency, intensity, and duration of attacks. We discuss the mechanisms of action of all medications and review potential side effects. Patients often want to know how long they will need to take medication, and we explain our philosophy to them.

Specifically, if patients' attacks occur with reduced frequency over a 4- to 6-month period, we being to taper the dosage of medication to find the lowest dose required for maintenance of adequate control or to discontinue medication entirely. If the attack frequency of migraine is reduced to two episodes per month with excellent response to acute care medication, then preventive medication will not be required. This may even occur with an attack frequency that is higher, provided that patients get prompt relief and experience minimal side effects with acute care medications. On the other hand, patients who have one 4-day episode per month that is completely unresponsive to acute care medications often require preventive medication.

Finally, when migraine does explode into a severe headache, we prescribe medication to terminate the attack pain and associated symptoms as quickly as possible. We make certain that our patients understand the importance of keeping their headache calendars up to date (see Chap. 2), when and how to take the medication, how much to take, and the maximum frequency permitted. Patients are told that it is essential to notify us if they are exceeding their limits.

We urge physicians not to prescribe large amounts of abortive or symptomatic medications with unlimited refills. Initially, we suggest that you prescribe enough for a month at a time with no refills to ensure that patients are not overusing medication. As you become more familiar with your patient and as headache control improves, it may be appropriate to authorize a larger supply or a refillable prescription. At the very maximum, sufficient medication to last between follow-up visits should be given. If patients run out of medication, they or the pharmacist will have to call your office at reasonable times for refills. Checking charts for refill patterns enables you to recognize overuse syndromes, noncompliance, or inadequate control.

Many materials are available to facilitate ongoing patient education and compliance. The American Council for Headache Education (ACHE) is a nonprofit foundation that provides a variety of supportive services and helps to establish support groups throughout the country. Support groups help patients recognize that they are indeed not alone. The National Headache Foundation (NHF) is also an excellent resource. ACHE can be reached at 1-800-255-ACHE, and NHF at 1-800-843-2256.

To paraphrase Roter and Hall, the physician should provide adequate information, so that patients have very few questions at the end of the initial consultation.

Diagnosis. Tell the patient your diagnosis and why you believe it is correct. You might use the International Headache Society criteria in your diagnosis and review them with patients for each of the primary headache disorders. If you believe that organic factors are involved, explain your impression to your patient and be as reassuring as possible.

Etiology. Explain the pathophysiology of headache as we currently understand it. Essentially, we explain to patients that headaches may be divided into two major areas: primary and secondary headache disorders. The *secondary headache disorders* are those that are symptomatic of an underlying medical problem that may be as ominous as tumors, hemorrhages, strokes, or aneurysms or more benign and attributable to allergy, sinus, or dental problems.

We then tell patients that the overwhelming majority (more than 90%) of patients with recurrent or chronic headache have one or more of the *primary headache disorders*: migraine, tension-type, or cluster headache. We review with our patients the current understanding of the pathophysiology of their headaches. We discuss the role of blood vessels and muscles and briefly explain the central mechanisms of migraine and the role of neurotransmitters or "chemical messengers" that are at play in these disorders. This is important because it validates the "real" nature of the pain and your understanding that it is not "psychological."

We find that patients can grasp the essential issues in the controversy as to whether or not migraine and tension-type headache are distinct or related disorders. Adequately explaining the pathophysiology gives patients a context in which to place your pharmacological and nonpharmacological treatment recommendations. This understanding improves compliance because it helps your strategy make sense to your patients.

Prognosis. Be sure to discuss the degree to which your patients' headaches are serious and explore the impact on his or her life. Further, your reviewing the history from your perspective—recapitulating the duration of illness and reviewing patients' therapeutic expectations—helps patients feel that you hear what they say and gives them an opportunity to clarify where necessary. We make it a point to tell our patients that it is not possible to cure any of the primary headache disorders but that a propensity to getting headaches may go into remission. It is important to reassure patients that in spite of the fact that headaches cannot be cured, they can and should expect **greater control, decreased frequency of headache, and enhanced quality of life.** This involves a mutually agreed upon plan of action for treatment.

Treatment. Patients should have a clear, specific understanding of your treatment plan when they leave your office and should use headache calendars to record in detail all abortive and preventive medications as well as nonpharmacological interventions that they use.

One of the most difficult problems on initial consultation and at ensuing visits revolves around the treatment of overuse syndromes. Patients who overuse analgesics and abortive medications are neither drug addicts nor substance abusers; they are either in pain or are anticipating pain or disability. These patients are trying to function optimally at all times. Understandably, many are frightened and some are terrified at the prospect of discontinuing their daily analgesics or ergotamines as recommended. We explain that the prognosis for patients who continue the overuse cycle is poor, at best. It is important to forewarn of probable short-term suffering, offset by long-term gain. The treatment of rebound is reviewed here and in Chapter 6.

In summary, off-the-shelf analgesics may be discontinued abruptly. We may use nonsteroidal anti-inflammatory medications on a tid basis with meals for 5 days, bid for 5 days, and qd for 5 days, or we may use isometheptene (Midrin) in the same manner. Patients must discontinue prn. medication for mild and, if possible, moderate headaches and should be reassured that medication will be provided for their most severe attacks. Opiates may be tapered slowly, perhaps with the use of clonidine 0.05 to 0.1 mg bid or tid to help suppress withdrawal symptoms.

Patients who take substantial amounts of these medications may require inpatient care, including intravenous therapy with dihydroergotamine (D.H.E. 45), which works best in an interdisciplinary setting. Because the danger of provoking seizures during barbiturate withdrawal is greater than that associated with withdrawal from any other type of medication, patients who take large or frequent doses of barbiturates should be considered for hospital admission for the initial withdrawal period. We recommend that patients withdrawing from medication be monitored more regularly than other patients, with follow-up visits every 2 weeks or as required.

Medications. Every patient should have a clear understanding of what medications to take, why they have been prescribed, how they work, and what potential effects and side effects may occur. Patients must know exactly how and when you want them to use the medications you have prescribed for them.

Scheduling medication dosage with respect to intervals between doses and meals can be tricky. Patients should receive explicit written instructions that are the same as those on prescription forms, bottles, and their daily headache calendars. Everything you do to reinforce your instructions enhances compliance.

Tests. If you order any diagnostic tests, you should carefully explain what you expect these tests to reveal and how the results will help you to manage the headaches more effectively. You should describe the testing environment and preparations that may be required. Be certain that patients who may require magnetic resonance imaging are not claustrophobic; if this is the case, consider referral to an open magnet facility and giving a small dose of benzodiazepine (5 mg diazepam) prior to imaging.

Life-Style. It is important not only to make recommendations for appropriate nutrition, exercise, sleep, alcohol intake, and smoking, but to clearly review those difficulties patients may expect in making these changes. Patients should understand that a period of weeks may elapse before the results of their efforts become evident. Determine whether patients are resistant to following these recommendations and, where appropriate, refer them to professionals (such as a nutritionist or exercise physiologist) to enhance compliance.

The last step in an initial consultation is to ask patients if they have any questions or concerns to discuss before they leave your office.

PARTICIPATION

Patient participation in treatment is one of the most important aspects of behavioral medicine. The external versus internal *locus of control* issue is critical. Patients with an external locus of control do not participate actively in their own treatment. Rather, they present with a passive attitude and an expectation that the doctor will "fix them" with a magic bullet or procedure. These patients have ongoing compliance problems and a poor prognosis if this position remains unchanged. Anything you can do to bring them to an internal locus of control is an improvement, and referral to experts in behavioral therapy may be highly beneficial. Patients with an internal locus of control are characterized by their active role in remediation of their own illnesses. Such a proactive position can be expressed by patients as: "What can I do to help myself?" or "I will take responsibility as well." Those patients who develop or present with an internal locus of control have a much better prognosis.

Headache calendars that enable patients to record frequency, intensity, and duration of pain and to identify potential trigger factors help to encourage patient participation.

Such self-monitoring of symptoms and medication intake as well as life-style changes automatically involve patients as active participants, and those patients who present with compliance issues should be counseled appropriately. Patients should fully understand their expectations and how to actively participate in a plan to reach them; they should also realize that without their active participation, therapeutic failure is likely. To this end, they must be educated to take responsibility for not running out of medication and for following a mutually agreed upon treatment plan.

Nonpharmacological Measures

Nonpharmacological therapies and approaches in the treatment of primary headache disorders are as varied as pharmacological therapies and are based on a theoretical understanding of factors that contribute to the pathogenesis of primary headache disorders and the mechanisms of action that underlie therapeutic interventions. Most headache specialists have concluded that a combination of pharmacological and nonpharmacological therapies is more effective than either one alone.

Traditionally, it has been more difficult to evaluate the validity of outcome data for nonpharmacological techniques because they embody so many variables and are virtually impossible to study under double-blind conditions. Clinicians who treat primary headache should be aware of available nonpharmacological modalities, so that they can recommend appropriate therapies and can react appropriately to patients' suggestions. For purposes of this discussion and review, we will divide the nonpharmacological therapies into *active* and *passive* approaches.

ACTIVE NONPHARMACOLOGICAL THERAPIES

Behavioral Medicine

Behavioral medicine is appropriate in treating any medical disorder and acknowledges the contribution of patients' behavior to both the development of illness and to its remediation. Unlike surgery or medication, behavioral medicine does not "do something" to patients. Rather, it assists patients in helping themselves and shifts the locus of control from an external source to an internal one. Specifically, it involves them in sharing responsibility for treatment.

For example, patients with coronary artery disease or chronic pulmonary disease who continue to smoke demonstrate destructive behavior that by definition interferes with the outcome of any treatment. In our practice, we have seen asthmatics who are under treatment with a variety of medications but who nonetheless continue to smoke. Patients who do not undertake appropriate life-style changes, such as exercising regularly, getting an appropriate amount of sleep, and stopping type A behavior, conduct themselves in a manner that is likely to adversely affect the outcome of treatment.

Just as diabetics must take responsibility for monitoring blood sugar and maintaining an appropriate diet, so must headache patients take appropriate measures that are likely to be beneficial. When compliance issues are evident, it is important that patients and physicians jointly review obstacles to compliance and discuss means of getting around them.

Behavioral medicine includes biofeedback, stress management, and relaxation exercises as well as modification of daily activities to achieve therapeutic effects. It relies upon a variety of techniques such as self-monitoring of medication intake, noting symptom frequency and intensity, logging of antecedents and consequences of symptoms, cognitive interventions, learning theory, and dietary intervention, all of which involve patients in shifting the locus of control from an external source to an internal one (themselves) and in sharing responsibility for treatment.

Biofeedback

To be properly understood, biofeedback must be viewed in the context of behavioral medicine. Biofeedback has a historical perspective more recently bought to fruition as a treatment modality because of the explosion of new technologies.

Biofeedback means biological or, perhaps more accurately, physiological feedback of information about biological processes. For example, the simplest and most common biofeedback technique occurs when a patient takes his or her temperature; the thermometer tells the specific degree of fever.

Biofeedback involves the use of instrumentation that reflects physiological processes of which the individual is not normally aware and which may be brought under voluntary control. These biological conditions include muscle tension, skin temperature, pulse amplitude, brain wave activity, galvanic skin response, skin potential response, blood pressure, heart rate, and others. Thus, biofeedback can increase individuals' ability to place physiological activities under voluntary control by providing information about these activities.

Neil Miller, a pioneer in the field, explained biofeedback with the analogy of a blindfolded golfer who could not see where the ball went and thus was unable to receive feedback or learn. Similarly, patients may not "see" changes in muscle tension or blood vessel activity; instrumentation can in effect remove the blindfold by providing information about these responses. Miller pointed out that Pavlov's work demonstrated that visceral responses can be modified by classical conditioning. Later human studies that used similar procedures demonstrated that changes in vasodilation, galvanic skin response, heart rate and rhythm, blood pressure, and salivation could be moved in a direction that was rewarded.

When patients are motivated, biofeedback can help improve their perception of biological processes. Generalization to their external world is also important. Behavioral medicine and biofeedback have been useful in a wide variety of psychophysiological and other disorders and should be properly administered and supervised by those with knowledge of behavioral medicine.

These techniques may be indicated in many of our headache patients, particularly those with tension-type headache; migraine, both with and without aura; and mixed headache disorders. Theoretical considerations, physiological precepts, and outcome studies point to efficacy in these disorders. Outcome data with cluster headache patients are not as promising; biofeedback is generally an inappropriate intervention for this disorder.

Since biofeedback relies heavily on an individual's ability to learn, it cannot be applied where that ability is sufficiently impaired. Thus, it is inappropriate for patients with organic or functional disorders, such as the schizophrenias with severe thought disorder, or in severely depressed patients with pervasive hopelessness or impaired concentration, cognition, and memory. Biofeedback can be more usefully applied after the depression or organic problem has been adequately treated.

Biofeedback is contraindicated in paranoid patients who may incorporate the instruments into a delusional system. Miller reminds us that reduction in motivation for being ill is a precondition if patients are to get better. From a behavioral viewpoint, the therapist must deal with the reinforcements that caused the symptom under treatment to be learned.

Biofeedback is commonly used in the treatment of tension-type headache and migraine in most headache centers in the United States. Electromyographic (EMG) feedback via the application of surface electrodes across the frontal muscles is the most commonly used type of biofeedback in tension-type headache. These surface electrodes measure discharge in muscle fibers. The raw electrical signal is then modified through the circuitry of the instrument, and the information is fed back to the patient via visual or auditory modes (lights that change color or audio tones that vary in pitch and frequency). Patients receive information related to levels of muscle activity. The threshold for feedback can be set and changed, such that EMG activity above the threshold level produces feedback and activity below the threshold level shuts off feedback. Computer software is now available to provide a variety of creative visual and audio feedback responses that show bio-

logical activity and graph patient progress over time.

Tension-type headaches are often associated with increased levels of muscle activity in frontal, temporal, trapezius, masseter, and other muscles. Some studies show muscle activity to be greater during headaches. Interestingly, patients with migraine show higher levels of muscle contraction than patients with tension-type headache. In addition, it is important to understand that many patients with tension-type headache do not have disorders of pericranial muscles. This raises the question as to the actual role of muscles (if any) in some cases of tension-type headache.

We believe that tension-type headache is a heterogeneous phenomenon that at times can be related to and caused by muscle contraction and at other times may be a product of central dysregulation of nociceptive mechanisms in the brain stem and elsewhere, similar to those involved in migraine. Interestingly, we have found in our own studies that patients with tension-type headache have an equal distribution of high EMG and normal or low EMG activity.

Those who support the musculogenic or peripheral theories of tension-type headache might argue that patients with low EMG readings may have had such prolonged activity of muscle contraction that they are no longer able to generate clinically significant levels of EMG activity. Those who advocate a central position would state that this normal or low activity speaks to central mechanisms as being paramount.

On the other hand, when normal controls are measured, the same distribution of high and low EMG activity is found. Prospective studies have not yet been done on patients prior to the development of headaches to determine whether changes in EMG activity occur once headaches develop. Thus, patients with no headache who demonstrate high levels of EMG activity may in theory subsequently report pain if central mechanisms are compromised. Furthermore, variables other than muscle contraction alone influence head pain. Keep in mind that muscle contraction is a reflexive response to pain anywhere in the body; even in patients with high levels of muscle activity who report pain, that activity may be a reaction to centrally generated pain rather than the etiologic cause of the pain. Nonetheless, successful biofeedback treatment can lower levels of autonomic arousal and appears to reduce pain levels for many patients.

In patients in whom EMG activity is high, the application of biofeedback is directed to train them to reduce contraction of involved musculature. Training increases patient awareness of frontal muscle activity and teaches them how to reduce it.

A variety of relaxation techniques and strategies help to achieve desirable responses. These usually start with deep, rhythmic, diaphragmatic breathing. Most patients are unaware that their breathing is superficial, with greater movement of their chests than of their diaphragms. Relaxation techniques may include suggestions that patients think of inhaling relaxation and exhaling tension; progressive relaxation techniques, alternating contraction and relaxation of skeletal muscles; autogenic training, which includes series of phrases repeated over and over again suggesting changes in the body such as warmth and heaviness; relaxation response; quieting response; and a variety of other techniques that may involve meditation or self-hypnosis.

Most frequently, patients attend sessions once per week, and less frequently twice weekly, up to a total of eight to 20 visits. During this time, they keep records of headache frequency, intensity, and duration; they also record details of home practice sessions and results. The goal, over time, is reduction in symptoms, the eventual elimination of the need for feedback via instrumentation, and the ability to generalize responses learned in the clinic setting to the outside world under normally stressful stimulus conditions. All of this must occur in carefully planned steps in a context of short-term achievable goals.

Budzynski and colleagues' studies in 1970 showed biofeedback to be effective in 70% of a headache population. Our colleagues Steve Baskin and Randy Weeks, at The New England Institute for Behavioral Medicine in Stamford, Connecticut, teach their patients

how to do a body scan. Patients learn to look for signs of tension in the muscles of the head, neck, shoulders, arms, and jaw and to recognize when they create muscle tension by hunching their shoulders and clenching their fists.

As patients become more aware of these usually unconscious activities, they can apply mini exercises for 1 to 2 minutes several times throughout the day. These include the breathing techniques and some of the relaxation responses discussed earlier. Patients who are involved in occupations that require a fixed position are told to get up every hour or so to practice techniques for reducing muscle tension.

Although both electromyographic and temperature training may be useful for either tension-type headache or migraine, as both techniques reduce autonomic activity, temperature training has traditionally been used for treatment of migraine (Fig. 7–2). Some of the initial applications of thermal training were introduced by Sargent and co-workers (1973), who reported that 63% of their migraine patients so trained experienced improvement in their conditions. Extracranial vascular changes during migraine attacks consist of increased temporal pulse amplitude and vasoconstriction of end arteries in the extremities. The usual presentation during a migraine attack is "cold hands and hot head." This reflects increased blood flow to the extracranial vasculature and decreased blood flow to the extremities. Since superficial skin temperature is in part a function of the volume of blood flow to the area, blood flow and skin temperature tend to change at the same time. When blood vessels are dilated, skin temperature increases; vasoconstriction is accompanied by decreases in skin temperature.

Information about vasomotor changes can be fed back to patients via a superficial thermistor that detects changes in skin temperature. Influences on vasomotor activity include external temperature of the surrounding environment, dietary factors such as caffeine, stress, medication, and psychological factors that trigger autonomic arousal. Some studies have even demonstrated a correlation between regional cere-

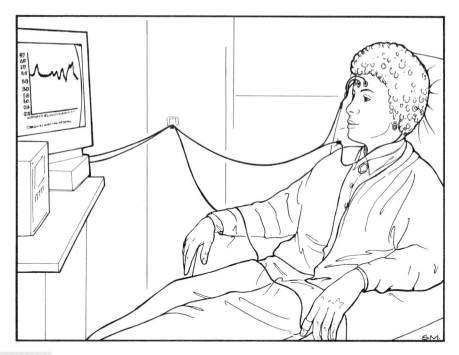

Figure 7–2

A patient undergoing electromyographic biofeedback training for frontal muscle relaxation as well as hand temperature biofeedback training.

bral blood flow and hand temperature, suggesting that even intracranial flow is influenced by peripheral skin temperature.

Thus, biofeedback training accompanied by autogenic and relaxation techniques teaches patients to raise hand temperature. Most studies on skin temperature demonstrate that migraine pain decreases as skin temperature rises. Some investigators believe that positive results from biofeedback occur as a result of decreased sympathetic tone secondary to retraining of the autonomic nervous system.

Hand warming, as the technique has been called, is more difficult to learn for physiological reasons than EMG activity reduction and thus is more tedious; treatment may be protracted. Migraine patients keep symptom logs or calendars, and do practice sessions in the same manner as do those with tension-type headache. Many patients are taught to control EMG activity first, followed by thermal training.

Patients with migraine with aura who have a warning may do especially well with these techniques when they use them at the onset of aura. Patients with migraine with-

out aura have a more difficult time aborting attacks because by the time they recognize the attack, it has already begun. Age may be a factor in outcome; some studies show treatment to be more effective in those under 30 and less so in those over 50; we have observed that children do considerably better than adults.

Cognitive Therapy

Cognitive therapy emphasizes the role of negative thoughts and irrational belief systems and their influence on feeling or affective states and behavior. For example, cognitive therapists may view depression in large part as an affective state that comes about as a result of negative feelings and cognitive distortions.

Others see cognitive distortions as a symptom of underlying depression. Today, studies on the treatment of depression demonstrate that the most favorable results are achieved with a combination of cognitive and pharmacological therapies. Comorbidity is discussed in Chapter 8. For the purposes of this discussion, however, it should be noted that patients with frequent migraine, and particularly those with chronic daily headache, have a higher incidence of comorbid depression and anxiety disorders.

Many individuals without overt depression may have a negative view of themselves and the world in which they live. These individuals view the glass as being half empty. Perhaps their hopelessness and skepticism about the future and success of treatment is based on previous failures and a history of living with intractable pain.

Cognitive therapy focuses on identifying negative statements and automatic thoughts such as "I will never get better," "I will always have these headaches," and "Nothing helps." Having these thoughts frequently may culminate in a self-fulfilling prophecy. Cognitive therapy is based on the hypothesis that a changed thinking style can alter associated feelings. Those well versed in cognitive therapy provide very direct and practical guidelines and a variety of tools and homework whose goals are to bring about change.

Type A patients (intense, competitive, time-urgent, impatient) who seek out frenetic environments are especially responsive to cognitive and behavioral therapy when they are motivated to produce change and are made aware of the destructive consequences of their behavior. These individuals "work at work and work at play."

Headache patients as a rule tend to be more accepting of biofeedback and cognitive therapy than they are of psychotherapy.

Psychotherapy

Physicians too frequently suggest psychotherapy out of frustration at patients' lack of response to treatment. It's a natural response; when we reach the end of our rope, we assume there must be something psychological at play. Not only is this not always the case, but the major reason for refractoriness to treatment is failure to address the overuse of acute care medications. Remember, too, that epilepsy, Parkinson's disease, and Huntington's chorea, among others,

were once considered psychological in origin. Thus, referral for psychotherapy should be based on more than the apparent exclusion of organic etiology. Ziegler has stated (personal communication), "It should certainly not be assumed that severe headaches that are intractable to various treatments are evidence of a deep-seated psychiatric disturbance."

If there is evidence of emotional disturbance contributing to, accompanying, or resulting from the headache disorder, then patients should be referred for psychotherapy as an adjunct to treatment. In no case should this referral convey a message that a psychotherapy referral represents discontinuation of "medical" treatment or interest or that the psychiatrist is the last and only hope of recovery. Rather, the referral should be made to address comorbid behavioral problems, depression, anxiety disorders, or personality disorders.

Physicians who are not psychiatrists should not underestimate their ability to provide supportive psychotherapy for headache in the form of simple reassurance, explanation of headache mechanisms, education, and permission to verbalize sources of stress in the environment. For example, simply asking patients to *describe a typical day* may go a long way in providing insight as to contributory behaviors and situations. Such discussion may be followed by some advice or suggestions for constructively dealing with and reducing stressful environmental factors. Many patients do not perceive that they are overextended or that they try to function in an excessively demanding environment. We often tell patients that the opposite of being selfish is being selfless. It may be useful to ask patients to get out their appointment books and to *schedule appointments to spend time on themselves*. This is followed by the suggestion that they keep that appointment and be on time just as they would for any other commitment.

For patients in whom psychological issues such as major depression and anxiety interfere with functioning, psychotherapy with a psychiatrist or psychologist who understands the biological mechanisms involved in pain and headache may be indicated.

Psychotherapeutic models include:

1. Individual psychotherapy, which may be psychoanalytical, psychodynamic, cognitive, or behavioral. Referring physicians should be familiar with therapists' orientation.

2. Family and/or conjoint therapy when there are clear-cut family-focused or marital issues. Some therapists specially trained in family therapy have an orientation that is conducive to producing meaningful change.

3. Group psychotherapy; support groups are invaluable, particularly for chronic headache patients, because they let patients know they are not alone and that others struggle with similar issues. Patients who attend support groups may learn helpful techniques from other members; however, support groups in which patients primarily complain about pain and the treatments they receive are not constructive. The most frequent complaints among headache patients revolve around physicians who seem uninterested, who place headache patients in some psychological wastebasket, and who do not provide sufficient time to review patients' questions and concerns.

The American Council for Headache Education provides support to support groups in many areas throughout the United States. ACHE National Headquarters can advise as to the availability of such groups. Alternatively, physicians may want to suggest that patients form a local group.

The goals of psychotherapy are to assist patients in achieving insight as to how conflict and anxiety may relate to somatic symptoms and to help patients find appropriate and constructive ways to address these issues. Patients learn to replace maladaptive responses with adaptive ones. Although there have been anecdotal reports of psychotherapeutic success, psychotherapy alone has not been demonstrated to ameliorate headache as well as combined approaches.

Exercise

The proper amount of appropriate exercise has been reported useful in decreasing chronic headache. Some studies have reported decreased frequency of both tension-type headache and migraine after patients institute programs of regular, moderate aerobic exercise. This decreased headache frequency may be the result of decreasing autonomic arousal through discharge of blocked sympathetic activity or of elevating levels of endorphins as demonstrated by Appenzeller in his study of wilderness runners (personal communication).

Nutrition

Nutritional considerations may be important for some patients, although widespread efficacy of dietary modification has not been established. We find that evaluation of caffeine intake and restricting or eliminating it are beneficial in the majority of our tension-type and migraine headache patients. Although caffeine may be helpful during a headache, excessive use can result in more headache, caffeinism, rebound phenomena, and increased anxiety. When you take a history of caffeine intake, include not only coffee and colas, but also less obvious items such as the caffeine content of prescription and nonprescription medication.

Most studies demonstrate that of all the various food triggers described in migraine, alcohol leads the list in its ability to provoke attacks. Eliminating foods that contain large amounts of vasoactive substances such as tyramine, phenylethylamine, and various nitrites may be helpful with some patients. Some studies have stated that this type of elimination diet may help only 10% of the migraine population. Nevertheless, a sufficient number of patients tell us that certain foods always trigger their migraine, so we find this consideration useful in headache management. Patients should be made aware that it is *chemical sensitivities* to the vasoactive components of certain foods rather than true food allergies that are at issue.

Patients may be more sensitive to certain foods during the time around their menses than at other times of the month. Dietary factors are discussed in more depth in Chapter 4. Many patients have found that the elimination of caffeine, meat, lactose-containing foods, and dairy products have contributed to a decrease in their headache frequency. NutraSweet (aspartame) has been reported to increase migraine frequency in up to 50% of patients. The makers of NutraSweet refute this effect, but we nonetheless suggest that patients omit it from their diets. Monosodium glutamate (MSG) is often cited as a trigger factor for migraine as well.

A few practitioners have viewed migraine as an immunoglobulin-E–mediated allergy in the classic antigen/antibody sense and use skin or cytotoxic blood tests to look for offending antigens. Controlled studies have not supported such an etiology or a single-factor operant in migraine or tension-type headache. Many patients who come to our Center have previously undergone extensive and expensive evaluation for allergies and have not benefited from such an approach. In fact, some have been placed on such restrictive regimens that there is little left for them to eat. Some studies in Great Britain demonstrated an 80% decrease in frequency of migraine when lactose-containing dairy products were eliminated, but these results have not been replicated in the United States.

PASSIVE NONPHARMACOLOGICAL THERAPIES

Passive techniques are those in which patients are not actively involved in their own treatment but rather are passive recipients.

Acupuncture

A traditional form of medicine in China, acupuncture has its roots in the Stone Age. Evidence for its effectiveness was originally empirical and anecdotal, but recent, more controlled studies suggest potential efficacy. The 1000 or so acupuncture points are divided into 12 major groups, each of which relates to an internal organ. Those points associated with the same organ are con-

nected by lines known as meridians. Studies indicate that these points demonstrate low resistance and high conductivity and can be identified with a skin resistance meter.

The Chinese see all of nature as a balance between the two opposing forces of the Yin and the Yang. A disturbance in this balance leads to disease. The Yin is female, passive, and restful. Headache is a Yang disorder and is thus treated by stimulating Yin points. It is interesting that headache, which predominates in women, is considered Yang.

Each acupuncture meridian is classified as either Yin or Yang, and stimulation may strengthen or weaken a particular meridian. Yin can be equated with parasympathetic tone and Yang with sympathetic. Explanations that seek to explain why acupuncture is effective have been based on the gate theory of pain, an overloading of pain-transmitting neurons. In fact, acupuncture may increase the production of adrenocorticotropic hormone (ACTH) and endorphins, and it has been shown that acupuncture analgesia can be reversed by naloxone, an opiate inhibitor. Some have said that acupuncture points and trigger points are identical.

Needles are manipulated by the acupuncturist to achieve the desired result (Fig. 7–3). When applied correctly, patients feel minimal to no pain or discomfort. The technique has gained wider acceptance in the West; some believe it may be enhanced by applying small electrical currents to the needles (electroacupuncture). Most acupuncture therapists agree that the technique, whichever is used, is ineffective if no response to treatment occurs within eight to 10 sessions.

Acupressure is a derivative of this technique. For migraine headache, patients may be taught to compress the web space of the hand ipsilateral to the headache with the thumb and forefinger of the opposite hand. For tension-type headache, the acupressure points that have been reported as helpful are just lateral to the orbits and on either side in the occiput.

Physical Therapy

Physical therapy has a long history; heat and massage have been used as muscle re-

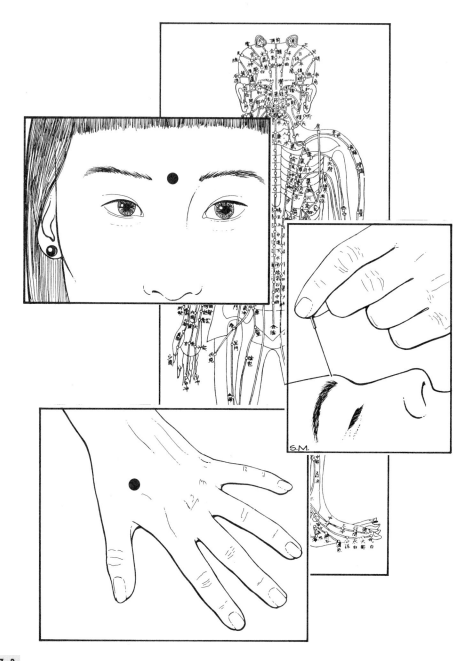

Figure 7–3

A patient undergoing acupuncture treatment for the relief of headache. Note the special acupuncture points between the eyebrows and in the web space of the hand. The meridians that connect these points are seen in the background.

laxants since antiquity. Physical therapy has been used to treat cervicogenic headache, a unilateral disorder that is triggered by certain movements of the neck. Modalities such as ultrasound, massage, and electrical stimulation have benefited patients with tension-type headache who demonstrate marked tightening, spasm, and tenderness on examination of the trapezius, occipitalis, and paracervical musculature.

The usual techniques we recommend involve increasing range of motion, improving posture, and performing specific exercises that stretch and strengthen cervical muscles.

We prefer techniques that patients can employ on their own.

Osteopathic Manipulative Therapy

Some patients' headaches respond favorably to osteopathic manipulation. Osteopathic physicians attend 4 years of medical school and receive training in anatomy, physiology, and manipulation. Osteopathic manipulation may be more effective in patients who manifest an external locus of control.

Chiropractic Therapy

Chiropractic therapy remains a controversial approach because of concerns over aggressive manipulation of the neck and its potential negative consequences. Chiropractic is based on the theory that all disease is caused by misalignment of vertebrae, resulting in pressure on adjacent somatic and sympathetic nerves. Once the pathology has been identified, treatment is geared toward structural realignment through the use of manual techniques known as "adjustments." The frequency of visits may vary from daily to twice weekly or less, and treatment may continue for long periods of time. In spite of the controversy among medical doctors, many patients report that chiropractic treatments have provided relief, and chiropractic remains a popular alternative to traditional medicine. If patients' headache pain is unrelieved in eight to 10 sessions, it is unlikely that further treatment will be helpful.

Massage Therapy

Massage therapy certainly may be included under the rubric of physical therapy, but some patients seek licensed individuals who practice only medical massage. Patients with tension-type headache who clearly demonstrate spasm, tightness, and tenderness of their cervical muscles may benefit from these techniques. A variety of massage techniques can provide relief.

Nerve Blocks

Nerve blocks may be helpful in the treatment of headache. The greater and lesser occipital nerves that supply the area of the skull from just below the occiput to the vertex and also behind the ear may be involved in the generation of head pain. We consider performing these blocks when there is extreme tenderness on palpation of the nerves in the suboccipital areas with radiation of the pain over or through the skull to the eye. The upper cervical roots (C2-3) enter the cord, synapse in the trigeminal nucleus caudalis, and provide the connections for the electrical activity to ascend to the central connections of the fifth nerve in the pons. It is via this pathway that pain may be referred to the orbits.

Although there is still much controversy about the pathophysiology of occipital neuralgia, injection of the occipital nerve has been reported by Anthony (1985) to abort cluster headache. Other investigators have reported successful termination of a migraine attack with occasional longer-term benefit. A local anesthetic, sometimes in combination with steroids, is injected below the occipital protuberance just lateral to the midline via a small-bore needle (Fig. 7–4). When successful, the results are generally dramatic and occur within minutes. The procedure may have to be repeated two or three times over several weeks; the effect may be cumulative.

Trigger Point Injections

Trigger point injections are based on the knowledge that some pain may be the result of myofascial disease. Travell and Simons (1983) and others observed that multiple points in the muscles throughout the body are painful to palpation and produce pain and twitching in the affected muscle.

In some headache patients, palpation of the appropriate trigger point will reproduce

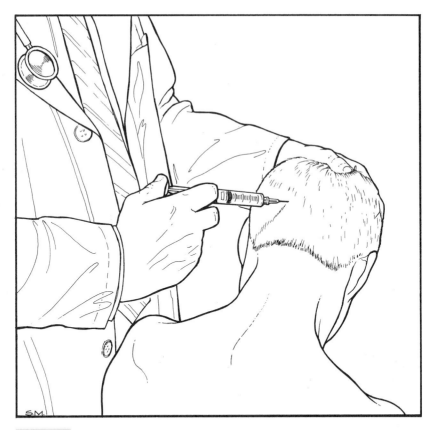

Figure 7–4

A patient undergoing a greater occipital nerve block for the treatment of occipital headache.

their usual pain. Trigger points for head pain may be located in the trapezius, paracervical, and sternocleidomastoid muscles. Dr. Travell has identified the various locations of these points as well as their referral sources. Treatment generally consists of the use of a needle to break up small fibrous bands in the muscle, thereby disrupting the pathology; it may entail the use of a small quantity of anesthetic such as lidocaine (Fig. 7–5). The treatment may also include spraying the muscle with a coolant such as ethyl chloride and stretching it to remove the source of pain. People with this condition usually have multiple trigger points, which require repeat treatments.

Transcutaneous Electrical Nerve Stimulation (TENS)

Transcutaneous electrical nerve stimulation has been explored for its application to headache. We have not been impressed with the effectiveness of TENS for head pain, although it may be effective for other types of chronic pain such as low back pain. The technique is a noninvasive outgrowth of dorsal column stimulators and is thought to have a theoretical basis in Melzack and Wall's gait theory of pain. Electrodes are placed between "pain and brain," thus stimulating impulses along large myelinated C fibers and thereby closing the "gate." This activates cells in the substantia gelatinosa in the dorsal horn of the spinal cord, in turn inhibiting target cells of small fibers that transmit pain impulses from the periphery (see Fig. 4–6). None of the traditional TENS units have been consistently effective in the treatment of head pain, and application to the head is dangerous for some patients. (TENS may induce smooth muscle contraction that could result in vasospasm of the carotid artery.)

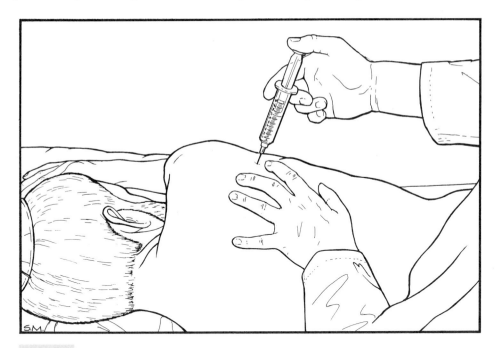

Figure 7–5

A patient undergoing a trigger point injection into a muscle that is producing radiation of pain to the head.

Solomon and Gugliemo, in a published study in 1985, used a nontraditional TENS unit, the Pain Suppressor, which is safe for application to the head. He found that it was more effective than placebo when used at a high enough strength to be perceived. Studies of the Liss Stimulator are ongoing; results are not yet available. Anecdotal reports and open studies suggest that further controlled studies are warranted.

Vitamins, Amino Acids, Herbs, and Trace Elements

The use of mega-vitamin therapy and trace element replacements has not been demonstrated to be effective in the treatment of headache; no double-blind, controlled studies of large samples are available. Anecdotally, we have found that 50 to 100 mg of vitamin B-6 and 400 U of vitamin E daily may be of some benefit in some headache patients. Schoenen and colleagues (1994) published a study demonstrating the efficacy of 400 mg per day of vitamin B-2 (riboflavin) in migraine. As stated earlier, large

dosages of vitamin A may in fact cause headache and contribute to the development of benign intracranial hypertension.

Magnesium has been studied by Mauskop and associates (1995) and may be beneficial in some 40 to 50% of patients. Studies by Ramadan and associates (1989) have demonstrated low intracellular magnesium in the migrainous brain. We suggest using Slo-Mag starting at 64 mg bid and increasing the dose to 128 mg bid. The major side effect, when present, is diarrhea, but it may be useful in patients who are constipated as a side effect of preventive headache medications.

Amino acids such as phenylalanine and tryptophan have also been studied without consistent results. Tryptophan is no longer available; a contaminated batch caused the eosinophilia-myalgia syndrome, resulting in great morbidity and some deaths among affected individuals.

A variety of herbs have been reported useful in migraine, the most popular of which is feverfew. Feverfew (see Chap. 6) is a member of the chrysanthemum family and has been used in England to prevent migraine. Although a recent study in Israel found no difference between feverfew and placebo in preventing headache, there is anecdotal evidence of its effectiveness.

Garlic, ginger, and ginseng have also been reported to be helpful in treating migraine, again, without scientific evidence. Fish oil, via a proposed mechanism of decreasing platelet agglutination, has also been used in the treatment of migraine.

More recently, a product known as Aqualyte or H2O+, consisting of hyper-oxygenated, potassium-enriched, magnesium-poor water, was discovered accidentally as a remedy for headache in Florida. Again, the evidence is anecdotal, although recent information from the manufacturer suggests that double-blind tests were scheduled to begin soon at a "leading school of medicine."

Naturopathy and Homeopathy

Both of these disciplines have been pursued by patients as alternatives to traditional medicine and may be sought out initially by patients who wish to avoid potential side effects of traditional pharmacological therapies or by patients for whom traditional treatments have failed to provide relief. *Naturopathy* uses only natural substances in minute amounts to provide a "healthier" balance of internal chemistry. *Homeopathy* differs in that the active ingredients in certain medications are used in addition to naturally occurring substances. These active substances are used in minute dosages that would be viewed in traditional medicine as ineffectual.

Conclusion

Nonpharmacological approaches run the gamut of A to Z: Acupuncture to Zen meditation. None of them helps all patients all the time, but some may be helpful to some of our patients some of the time. This is equally true of traditional medical approaches. It is important to keep an open mind and to evaluate not only traditional therapies but alternative therapies as well. The Hippocratic oath reminds us to "do no harm" and indeed some of these therapies will not harm patients medically or economically and should not be rejected out of hand. We should operate as guides and express our opinions and experience, but it is important to allow patients to make the final judgment. As responsible practitioners, we have a duty to steer patients away from radical treatments such as changing all dental fillings, the use of large amounts of questionably effective substances, inappropriate surgical intervention, and unusually restrictive dietary programs.

Finally, we should not forget a time-proven nonpharmacological approach to migraine: sleep and an ice-pack. There are several good theoretical mechanisms by which cold might work. Several devices are helpful in application of cold, including the headache ice-pillow developed at the California Medical Clinic for Headache. The application of cold may work by constricting blood vessels, reducing muscle spasm, or overriding electrical impulses in afferent pain pathways. Cold works best in the frontotemporal area, over the eyes, and over the nape of the neck.

Although there is much we have learned about primary headache disorders, we have a long way to go in uncovering the full story and discovering improved pharmacological and nonpharmacological therapies. The story of the three blind men and the elephant may help to summarize the current status on controversies between and among various disciplines. The blind man who feels the elephant's tail describes the elephant as being like a snake. The one who feels the leg describes the elephant as a broad tree trunk, and the one who feels the side of the elephant says, "No, the elephant is like a house." All three are a part of the story, but none represents the whole picture.

SUGGESTED READINGS

American Council for Headache Education: *Migraine: The Complete Guide.* New York: Dell Trade Paperbooks, 1994.

Anderson JAD, Basker MA, Dalton R: Migraine and hypnotherapy. *Int J Clin Exp Hypn.* 1975;23(1):48–58.

Andrasik F, Pallmeyer TP, Blanchard EB, et al: Continuous vs interrupted schedules of thermal biofeedback: An exploratory analysis with clinical subjects. *Biofeedback Self Regul.* 1984;9(3):291–8.

Andreychuk T, Skriver C: Hypnosis and biofeedback in the treatment of migraine headache. *Int J Clin Exp Hypn.* 1975;23(3):172–83.

Anthony M: Arrest of attacks of cluster headache by local steroid injection of the occipital nerve. In Rose, FC, ed, *Migraine: Clinical and Research Aspects.* Basel: Karger. 1985;169.

Appelbaum KA, Blanchard EB, Hillhouse JJ, et al: Treatment outcome in chronic vascular headache. *Biofeedback Self Regul.* 1988;13(1).

Arrowsmith, FA: Ongoing treatment considerations in the management of headache patients. In Rapoport AM, Sheftell FD, eds, *Headache: A Clinician's Guide to Diagnosis, Pathophysiology and Treatment Strategies.* Costa Mesa, CA: PMA Publishing Corp. 1993;235.

Bakal DA, Demjen S, Kaganov JA: Cognitive behavioral treatment of chronic headache. *Headache.* 1981; 21:81–86.

Bakal DA, Kaganov JA: Muscle contraction and migraine headache: Psychophysiologic comparison. *Headache.* 1977;17:208–15.

Benson H: *The Relaxation Response.* New York: Avon Books.

Benson H, Klemchuck HP, Graham JR: The usefulness of the relaxation response in the therapy of headache. *Headache.* 1974;14:49–52.

Blanchard EB, Andrasik F: Biofeedback treatment of vascular headache. In Hatch JP, Fisher JG, Rugh JD, eds, *Biofeedback: Studies in Clinical Efficacy.* New York: Plenum. 1987.

Blanchard EB, Andrasik F, Ahles TA, et al: Migraine and tension headache: A meta-analytic review. *Behav Res Ther.* 1980;11:613.

Blanchard EB, Appelbaum KA, Guarneri P, et al: Treatment outcome in chronic tension headache. *Biofeedback Self Regul.* 1988;13:57–8.

Budzynski TH, Stoyva JM, Adler CS: Feedback-induced muscle relaxation: Application to tension headache. *J Behav Ther Exp Psychiatry.* 1970;1:205–11.

Budzynski TH, Stoyva JM, Adler CS, et al: Headache: A controlled outcome study. *Psychosom Med.* 1973;35:484–96.

Burks SL: *Managing Your Migraine.* Totowa, New Jersey: Humana Press. 1994.

Chapman-Smith D: Chiropractic management of headache. *The Chiropractic Report.* 1991;5(2):1.

Crue BL (ed): *Chronic Pain.* New York: Spectrum Publications. 1979.

Diamond S, Medina JL: Value of biofeedback in the treatment of chronic headache: The patients' opinions. *Res Clin Stud Headache.* 1978;6:155–159.

Hondlor N: *Diagnosis and Nonsurgical Management of Chronic Pain.* New York: Raven Press. 1991.

Holroyd KA, Holm JE, Penzien DB, et al: Long-term maintenance of improvements achieved with (abortive) pharmacological and nonpharmacological treatments for migraine: Preliminary findings. *Biofeedback Self Regul.* 1988;14(4):301–308.

Holroyd KA, Penzien DB, Hursey KG, et al: Change mechanisms in EMG biofeedback training: Cognitive changes underlying improvements in tension headache. *J Consult Clin Psychol.* 1984;52:1039–1053.

Kohlenberg RJ, Cahn T: Self-help treatment for migraine headaches: A controlled outcome study. *Biofeedback Self Regul.* 1980;5(3):371–372.

Kurland HD: Treatment of headache pain with auto-acupressure. *Dis Nervous System.* 1979;37:137–139.

Lake AE, Rainey J, Papsdorf JD: Biofeedback and rational-emotive therapy in the management of migraine headache. *J Appl Behav Anal.* 1979;12:127–140.

Largen JW, Mathew RJ: Cerebral blood flow and headache activity in normal volunteers and migraineurs trained in skin temperature self-regulation. In Mathew RJ, ed, *Treatment of Migraine: Pharmacological and Biofeedback Considerations.* New York: Spectrum Publications. 1981.

Mathew NT: Prophylaxis of migraine and mixed headache: A randomized controlled study. *Headache.* 1981;21:105.

Mauskop A, Altura BT, Craco RQ, et al: Intravenous magnesium sulphate relieves acute migraine in patients with low serum ionized magnesium levels. *Neurology.* 1995;45(Suppl 4):A379.

Medina JL, Diamond SD: The role of diet in migraine. *Headache.* 1978;18:31.

Medina JL, Diamond S, Franklin MA: Biofeedback therapy for migraine. *Headache.* 1976;16:115–8.

Melzack R, Wall PP: Pain mechanisms: A new theory. *Science.* 1965;150:971.

Neuchterlein KH, Holroyd JC: Biofeedback in the treatment of tension headache. *Arch Gen Psychiatry.* 1980;37:866.

Packard RC: What does the headache patient want? *Headache.* 1979;19:370.

Pedersen SA, Golden RN, Evans DL, Haggerty J Jr: Neurobiological aspects of behavior. In Stoudmire A, ed, *An Introduction to Human Behavior.* Philadelphia: JB Lippincott Co. 1990;261.

Ramadan NM, Halvorson H, Vande-Linde A, et al: Low brain magnesium in migraine. *Headache.* 1989; 29:590.

Rapoport AM, Sheftell FD, eds. *Headache: A Clinician's Guide to Diagnosis, Pathophysiology and Treatment Strategies.* Costa Mesa, California: PMA Publishing Corp. 1993.

Rapoport, AM, Sheftell FD. *Headache Relief.* New York: Fireside. 1991.

Roberts AH: Behavioral management of headache. In Dalessio DD, Silberstein SD, eds, *Wolff's Headache and Other Head Pain,* 6th ed. New York: Oxford University Press. 1993;483.

Roter DL, Hall JA. *Doctors Talking with Patients/Patients Talking with Doctors.* Westport, CT: Auburn Health. 1992.

Sacks O: *Migraine: Understanding a Common Disorder.* Berkeley and Los Angeles: University of California Press. 1985.

Sargent JP, Green EE, Walters ED: Preliminary report on the use of autogenic feedback training in the treatment of migraine and tension headaches. *Psychosom Med.* 1973;35:129.

Sargent J, Solbach P, Coyne L, et al: Results of a controlled experimental outcome study of nondrug treatments for the control of migraine headaches. *J Behav Med.* 1986;9(3):291.

Schoenen J, Lenaerts M, Bastings E: High-dose riboflavin as a prophylactic treatment of migraine: Results of an open pilot study. *Cephalalgia.* 1994;14:328.

Solomon S, Gugliemo KM: Treatment of headache by transcutaneous nerve stimulation. *Headache.* 1985; 25:12.

Stevenson DD: Allergy, atopy, nasal disease, and headache. In Dalessio DD, Silberstein SD, eds, *Wolff's Headache and Other Head Pain*, 6th ed. New York: Oxford University Press. 1993;291.

Stroebel CF, Ford MR, Strong P, et al: *Quieting Response Training: Five-Year Follow-Up of a Clinical Biofeedback Practice*. Louisville, Kentucky: BSA. 1981.

Travell J, Simons DG: *Myofascial Pain and Dysfunction: The Trigger Point Manual*. Baltimore: Williams & Wilkins. 1983.

Turin A, Johnson WG: Biofeedback therapy for migraine headaches. *Arch Gen Psychiatry.* 1976;33:517–9.

Weeks, RE: Behavioral medicine approach to headache. In Rapoport AM, Sheftell FD, eds, *Headache: A Clinician's Guide to Diagnosis, Pathophysiology and Treatment Strategies*. Costa Mesa, CA: PMA Publishing Corp. 1993;215.

Welch KMA: Migraine: A biobehavioral disorder. *Arch Neurol.* 1987;44:323.

CHAPTER EIGHT

Psychiatric Aspects of Primary Headache Disorders

There is still much controversy over the origin of primary headache disorders. One of the most hotly debated issues is the relationship between psychological factors and headache. Few other disorders have been shrouded in as much myth and misconception as headache has. Some of the more common myths include "headache is all in your mind," and "stress is the primary reason some people have headaches and others do not."

The pathophysiology of primary headache disorders remained relatively obscure to most practicing physicians until the 1970s, when the earlier work of Harold Wolff and his colleagues and major advances in the field shed more light on neurobiological mechanisms. As with most disorders whose causes have been poorly understood, psychiatric causality has long been a convenient explanation. At one time, epilepsy, Parkinson's disease, Huntington's chorea, and other conditions were regarded as psychiatric in origin. Viewing primary headache disorders as psychologically caused based on negative neurological examina-

tions, computed tomographic and magnetic resonance imaging scans, and electroencephalograms did headache patients a grave disservice.

Central neurotransmitters, such as the biogenic amines (catecholamines and indolamines) and peptides (endorphins and enkephalins), which we now know play important roles in primary headache disorders, also play central roles in determining mood and behavior. Understanding these neurotransmitters and their specific mechanisms of action may also shed light on some of the theoretical and complex relationships between primary headache disorders and psychological symptomatology.

To understand the relationship between psychiatric factors and primary headache disorders from the clinician's point of view, it is best to define these relationships from three major perspectives: 1) etiological, 2) psychophysiological, and 3) comorbidity. An understanding of these perspectives can be very helpful in developing a cohesive approach to dealing with these issues in clinical practice.

Etiological Perspective

The earliest theories on the origin of headache were related to demonic possession and a variety of religious beliefs. This understanding of the "causes" of headache led to a variety of treatments that included religious rituals, trepanation, blood letting, and purges to rid patients of demons or bad humors. Some current theories that ascribe the etiology of headache to psychiatric factors include the following disorders.

PSYCHOGENIC PAIN DISORDERS

The term *psychogenic pain disorder*, as described in the third edition of the Diagnostic and Statistical Manual of Mental Disorders (DSM-III), implies that psychogenic pain is either not real or is somehow different from "organic pain." The term psychogenic continues to be used in a variety of ways and is usually understood as pain that is the result of psychological factors. Although psychological factors may contribute to and affect the course of primary headache disorders, a causal relationship should not be assumed. Even in cases in which psychogenicity may apply, the pain is just as real to the patient as pain stemming from organic or primary headache disorders. If the pain is not "real," as the term might suggest, what then is the patient experiencing? Perhaps the patient is interpreting normal sensory input as pain, but on the other hand, perhaps these psychogenic pain patients have some disregulation of central antinociceptive mechanisms; there is evidence to suggest that this might indeed be the case.

SOMATOFORM DISORDERS

Somatoform is the current replacement of the earlier term *psychogenic*, as described in the current version of DSM-IV. Briefly, a somatoform disorder is characterized by physical symptoms that suggest a physical disorder for which **no demonstrable organic findings** or known physiologic mechanisms exist and for which there is a strong presumption that symptoms are linked to psychological factors. Symptom production in these disorders is not intentional. Our psychiatric understanding of "somatization" is the process whereby the body or symptoms are used for psychological purposes such as primary (relief of anxiety) or secondary (gratification of dependency needs) gain. This can occur in the presence of demonstrable disease as well as in its absence. For example, symptoms may be amplified in order to gain attention. If a physician is not aware of all that we have learned about the neurobiology of primary headache disorders, a somatoform diagnosis may be mistakenly applied. The variety of somatoform disorders includes the following:

Somatization Disorder. This is characterized by a variety of physical complaints beginning prior to age 30 and associated with impairment in role functioning and the frequent seeking of medical treatment. The diagnosis is based on the presence of at least four pain symptoms, two gastrointestinal, one sexual, and one pseudoneurological (which suggests a neurological condition but is not limited to pain). In addition, the symptoms cannot be fully explained by a known medical condition, or, when there is a related condition, the physical complaints and role impairment are in excess of what one would expect. Symptoms are **not intentionally produced**.

Conversion Disorder. Conversion disorders generally present as the acute loss of function in the voluntary motor system or the special senses. Psychological factors are judged to be directly involved because of their close proximity to the onset of these deficits. As in somatoform disorders in general, the deficit is not intentionally produced and cannot be explained by a general medical problem. Conversion disorders may also result in distress or impairment in role functioning.

Somatoform Pain Disorder. Pain in one or more sites is the predominant focus and results in significant distress and functional impairment. Psychological factors are judged to be important in the onset, severity, and maintenance of pain.

Hypochondriasis. Here the key word is "preoccupation" with fears of having a serious disease, based on the person's misinterpretation of bodily symptoms. As a rule, patients who suffer with hypochondriasis maintain a vigil over all bodily functions, and any deviation from what they perceive as the norm heralds great distress. This preoccupation persists despite extensive medical evaluation and reassurance.

This preoccupation and belief that one has a disease is not of delusional intensity. Delusions are defined as "fixed false" beliefs based in reality. One of the best examples of the degree to which a delusion can be fixed is the patient who presents to a psychiatrist with the belief that he is dead. The psychiatrist asks, "Do dead people bleed?" And the patient responds, "Of course not!" The psychiatrist takes a sterile pin, pricks the patient's finger, and draws blood. The patient looks at his finger and calmly states, "I guess dead people **do** bleed!"

Patients with hypochondriasis do not have this degree of fixed false belief and they do respond, albeit temporarily, to reassurance. The duration of the disturbance is at least 6 months. All patients with acute illness may develop hypochondriacal symptoms in the sense that they are preoccupied and greatly concerned about their illness. Hypochondriacal complaints may be a presenting symptom of depression; it is important to watch for the usual symptoms of depressive illness.

OTHER PSYCHIATRIC DISORDERS

A rare type of psychiatric disorder, which may be linked causally to headache, is delusional disorder of the somatic type. Patients with such disorders present with persistent, bizarre, delusional complaints not caused by another mental disorder such as schizophrenia or mood disorders. These patients describe such bizarre causes of their pain as snakes crawling through their heads or beams penetrating their brains.

All of the disorders just described share the mechanism of **not being intentional.** The following two psychiatric disorders involve the conscious production of symptoms.

Malingering. This involves the intentional production of false symptoms motivated by external incentives such as financial compensation or avoidance of prosecution or military service. Malingering may also be seen in patients who seek narcotics in office and emergency room settings. A careful premorbid history may reveal factors such as antisocial behavior and irresponsibility. Secondary gain is usually obvious. Malingering is often invoked by attorneys opposing patients with post-traumatic headache who are involved in litigation. It is our experience that **malingering is rarely seen** in the headache patients, including those with post-traumatic headache.

Factitious Disorders. Factitious disorders also involve the intentional production of physical symptoms. However, the secondary gain is not as obvious as with malingering. Often the motivation is to seek and assume a sick role. The patient's energy may be directed toward admissions or extended stays in hospitals (eg, Münchausen's syndrome or factitious fever, the practice of putting the thermometer on the light bulb to raise the temperature reading). External incentives for this behavior are absent.

In summary, perhaps headache with etiological psychiatric factors should be classified as secondary headache disorders that are symptomatic of an underlying disorder, which in this case would be psychiatric. This classification would be consistent with that of other secondary headache disorders that are caused by organic factors such as tumor, hemorrhage, infection, or metabolic disorder.

"The Migraine Personality"

This concept, although not a psychiatric diagnosis, is worth mentioning because of its historical significance and the fact that it is often misused and misinterpreted. This term was originally coined by Harold Wolff of New York as a result of his review of clinical files. He described the migraine personality as rigid, perfectionist, controlled, orderly, tense, meticulous, ambitious, fearful of making mistakes, overly conscientious, and in need of winning approval. While it is certainly true that many migraine patients present with this constellation of traits, many others do not. Conversely, many patients with these personality characteristics do not suffer from migraine or any other type of primary headache disorder. More accurately, these characteristics may be ascribed to patients with an obsessive compulsive orientation or style.

Some physicians have mistakenly interpreted Wolff's work as indicating that personality factors are primary in causing the headache when indeed this was not his intention. However, those patients who do have a biological vulnerability and happen to present with obsessive compulsive characteristics or "Type A" characteristics, as defined by Meyer Friedman, may find that these behavioral patterns adversely influence the course of their disorder. In fact, Wolff called migraine a "biological reprimand" to patients whose migraine attacks followed periods when they were overextended. John Graham referred to migraine as "angina of the soul."

From the clinician's point of view, it is best not to suggest that an individual's personality style is the cause of their disorder but rather to educate the patient as to the adverse consequences of these behaviors superimposed on a foundation of biologic vulnerability. This attitude will be discussed further in the next section on psychophysiological considerations.

Psychophysiological Perspective

Psychophysiological disorders are defined as *objective* pathophysiological changes in end organs that are generally under the control of the autonomic nervous system, related to or aggravated by psychological factors. In DSM-III-R, migraine is classified under psychological factors affecting physical conditions and in DSM-IV under psychological factors affecting medical conditions.

The term **psychophysiological** has supplanted the older term *psychosomatic* and reflects a subtle differentiation in definition. Psychophysiological refers to mind/function and psychosomatic to mind/body. In the older nosologies, a section in DSM-II listed a variety of psychophysiological conditions by system (eg, cardiovascular, gastrointestinal, pulmonary). This has been eliminated from the DSM so as not to imply that disorders such as duodenal ulcer, ulcerative colitis, and asthma are psychiatric disorders by virtue of their inclusion in the manual.

At the same time, the current nosology reflects an attempt to address concerns about eliminating medical disorders that may reflect mind/body interactions by including the diagnosis of "psychological factors affecting medical conditions," with subsequent reference of the medical condition to the International Classification of Diseases, ninth edition. DSM-IV reflects concern by stating, "They may precipitate or exacerbate symptoms of a general medical condition by eliciting stress-related physiological responses (eg, causing chest pain in individuals with coronary artery disease or bronchospasm in those with asthma)." These criteria may be extended to similar factors which may **trigger** tension-type headache or migraine.

In our opinion, the major areas of intersection between psychological factors and primary headache disorders exist in the realm of psychophysiological interaction. In other words, we are dealing with a group of conditions in which a physiological disorder does exist and psychological factors play a role, although not necessarily causally, in their expression. It is most likely that individuals possess a level of genetic or neurochemical predisposition to migraine. The expression of attacks may then depend on a variety of factors, including environmental and personality ones as well as an individual's ability to adapt successfully to his or her environment.

When biological vulnerability is very high, perhaps even the normal stresses and strains inherent in daily living may result in significant symptomatology. When biological vulnerability is low, perhaps greater degrees of stress or more ineffective coping styles may be preconditions that provoke attacks. Again, this model is the most salient in assessing migraine and tension-type headache in that a variety of factors can trigger a biological vulnerability, including but not limited to the role of personality, behavioral styles, environmental challenges, and coping skills. Using this model, treatment approaches would be behavioral and would include cognitive therapies, biofeedback, stress management, and other strategies described previously.

Many investigators have studied the mind/body interaction, including Meyer, Bernard, Cannon, Gant, Pavlov, and Selye. It was Franz Alexander who wrote of psychosomatic illness as reflecting the very real presence of objective pathophysiology, not to be confused with the group of somatoform disorders, including hypochondriasis, in which objective pathophysiology is not present. Some of the earlier psychoanalytic theories of psychosomatic disorders reflected the understanding that the symptom was tied to a specific personality style. In other words, those with a dependent orientation might be more prone to disorders such as asthma or ulcer, and those with a more obsessive compulsive style would be more likely to present with symptoms such as ulcerative colitis or irritable bowel syndrome.

Alexander proposed that a variety of stimuli would give rise to an arousal pattern inherent in the organism, which would lead to a response if that arousal pattern were sustained. It is likely that an arousal pattern is genetically determined, although some investigators have suggested that conditioning may play a role as well.

To apply this model to migraine, a variety of internal or external "trigger" stimuli, including hormones, dietary factors, chronobiological changes, sensory stimuli, and "stress," would be required. The internal triggers specific to migraine patients may include spreading depression, activation of the trigeminovascular system, serotonergic dysregulation, and platelet agglutination. The resulting response would then be characterized by the migraine attack. Consider

stress, for example: When biological susceptibility is very high, the normal stresses and strains inherent in daily living might be sufficient to provoke occasional attacks in the absence of psychopathology or poor coping skills. When the vulnerability is lower, more severe or prolonged stressors or maladaptive responses would be required to provoke the attack.

When stressful factors in the environment are dealt with adaptively, the "stress" is resolved and may not be of great consequence. When the stress is prolonged or severe or responses are maladaptive, or a combination of these conditions exists, chronicity ensues, which may be an ongoing provocative factor contributing to increased frequency and constancy of headache.

Comorbidity Perspective

Just as the presence of migraine or tension-type headache does not "immunize" patients against developing organic causes of headache such as tumor, neither does it prevent patients from developing or suffering from other comorbid disorders such as depression, anxiety, or personality disorders. Thus, a variety of psychiatric diagnoses can be made independent of but along with migraine and tension-type headache or any other medical disorder.

We know from a biological perspective that the biogenic amines and neuropeptides appear to play key roles in the pathogenesis of primary headache disorders. Although multiple neurotransmitter mechanisms may be involved, there has been an intense focus on the role of serotonin both peripherally and centrally.

Serotonin is thought to play a critical role in a variety of disorders such as anxiety, depression, obsessive compulsive disorder, vasospasm, and eating disorders. In the comorbidity of headache and depression, the relationship between the two is more complex than one might think. For example, common sense would dictate that any person with chronic pain would also suffer from depression secondary to that pain. We know that pain and depression interact in a variety of ways. Not only may chronic pain lead to depression, but depression itself may lower the pain threshold and pain tolerance. Arguments continue about which comes first, but regardless of the final answer, clinicians must acknowledge both disorders and properly identify comorbid psychiatric diagnoses to render effective treatment.

Conversely, we know that headache is the most frequent somatic complaint in patients with major depression. Most psychiatric inpatient units have a standing order for acetaminophen two tablets every 4 to 6 hours as needed for headache. In addition, we know that patients with chronic daily headache present with a variety of depressive symptoms such as sleep disorders, appetite disturbances, decreased energy levels, decreased interest in activities, decreased libido, decreased ability to experience pleasure, and functional impairment. Further, stress and anxiety may increase the intensity of and functional impairment associated with any neurological condition, including Parkinson's disease and multiple sclerosis.

Many studies have examined the comorbidity of primary headache and psychiatric illness. Researchers such as Merikangas, Isler, and Breslow have addressed these from an epidemiological point of view and have shown that the lifetime prevalence of anxiety, phobia, and depression is significantly greater in patient with migraine than in non-migraine control groups. One-year prevalence studies of major depression in migraine have demonstrated a fourfold difference between major depression in migraine patients and non-migraine control subjects.

In a large cohort study, Merikangas and colleagues (1990) showed the combination of anxiety disorders and major depression to be significantly associated with migraine. Those studies indicated greater anxiety in childhood, migraine headache in adolescence and in the 20s, and depressive disorders in later life. A recent study by Breslow entitled "Migraine and Major Depression: A Longitudinal Study," presents the first body of evidence that indicates that each disorder increases the risk of onset of the other. Her findings favor the shared mechanism expla-

nation. In other words, it may not be that one causes the other, but rather shared neurobiological or psychobiological mechanisms underlie both.

It is important to identify all medical and psychiatric disorders that are comorbid with migraine. For example, clinicians must be aware of the comorbidity of asthma and headache to avoid using contraindicated medications such as β-blockers. Sumatriptan or ergotamine should not be administered to patients with coronary vasospastic disorders. These concepts are equally true in psychiatric comorbidity. Let us examine the important Axis I and Axis II disorders that may present comorbidly with primary headache disorders.

AXIS I DISORDERS

Axis I disorders, as defined in DSM-IV, are clinical syndromes such as major depression, schizophrenia, and alcohol dependency. Examples are:

1. Psychological Factors Affecting Medical Condition
2. Somatoform Disorders
3. Adjustment Disorders with Physical Complaints
4. Major Depression
5. Dysthymic Disorder
6. Delusional Disorders of the Somatic Type
7. Malingering
8. Factitious Disorders with Physical Symptoms
9. Anxiety Disorders

Several of these have already been discussed. We will outline briefly the major symptoms of the depressive and anxiety disorders.

Symptoms of Major Depressive Episodes

Symptoms associated with major depressive episodes include depressed mood, sadness or emptiness, markedly diminished interest or pleasure in most activities, significant weight loss or changes in appetite in the absence of dieting, sleep disturbances, psychomotor retardation or agitation, loss of energy or fatigue, feelings of worthlessness or guilt, decreased ability to concentrate or think clearly, severe indecisiveness, recurrent thoughts of death or recurrent suicidal ideation or plans.

These symptoms cause significant distress and impair role functioning. In interviewing patients, clinicians should use everyday language such as "Do you feel blue?" or "Do you feel sad a good deal of the time?" rather than "Are you depressed?"

It is essential to identify depression as a clinical syndrome because it has a high rate of morbidity and mortality and can be treated successfully. If the headache is addressed without diagnosis and treatment of the depression, headache treatment outcome will be severely compromised.

Dysthymia

Dysthymia is similar to major depressive symptoms but is less intense and lasts for at least 2 years. Patients with dysthymia tend to have a negative cognitive style, look at the glass as being half empty, and seem to have a cloud of gloom over their heads at all times.

Adjustment Disorders

In adjustment disorders, one sees the development of emotional and behavioral symptoms in response to an identifiable stressor occurring within 3 months of the onset of the stressor. This diagnosis requires that the distress is in excess of what would ordinarily be expected from exposure to the stressor. Patients with adjustment disorders may also demonstrate symptoms of anxiety or depression or both, but not of sufficient degree to fulfill the criteria for major depression or dysthymia.

Anxiety Disorders

These include panic disorders with or without agoraphobia and recurrent, unex-

pected panic attacks. For proper diagnosis, patients must develop four or more of the following symptoms, which reach a peak within 10 minutes: palpitations; tachycardia; sweating; trembling; sensations of shortness of breath, smothering, or choking; chest pain or discomfort; nausea or abdominal distress; dizziness; unsteadiness; light-headedness or faintness; derealization or depersonalization; fear of losing control or going crazy; fear of dying; paresthesias; and chills or hot flashes. The number of patients with overt panic disorders who have not been diagnosed is surprising. Other criteria for panic disorder includes anticipatory anxiety regarding future attacks, concerns about the implications of the attacks, and significant behavioral changes related to these attacks.

It is important to recognize anxiety disorders. When a diagnosis of a comorbid psychiatric condition is made, it is important to explain to patients that such a diagnosis does not mean that their headaches are the result of a psychiatric illness, but rather that they are accompanied by psychiatric symptoms. These symptoms can generally be treated in the domain of the primary care physician, internist, or neurologist. If treatment is unsuccessful, then appropriate psychiatric referral can be made in the context of educating the patient, as described in Chapter 7.

The major nonpharmacological approaches include cognitive and behavioral therapies; pharmacological approaches include the use of appropriate antidepressant medications that may be beneficial to patients with both anxiety and depressive disorders. In the past, imipramine (Tofranil) and phenelzine (Nardil) were commonly used, excellent medications for panic disorders; more recently, the specific serotonin reuptake inhibitors have become more popular. Long-term benzodiazepine use is best handled with appropriate psychiatric consultation.

AXIS II DISORDERS

Axis II disorders include developmental and personality disorders such as obsessive-compulsive disorder, hysterical personality disorder, and borderline personality disorder. The most difficult challenges are those patients who present with primary headache disorders in a climate of both Axis I and Axis II disorders, with the borderline personality representing the most severe challenge, not only to primary care physicians but to psychiatrists as well.

Borderline Personality Disorder

This personality disorder bears mentioning because it involves major compliance and behavioral problems as well as presenting serious challenges to the caregiver. The disorder is characterized by unstable relationships that alternate between over-idealization and devaluation. For example, borderline patients may tell you, their physician, that you are the best doctor they have ever consulted and that their search is finally over. No other doctor has listened as intensively or appears to be as interested, and they know that the future is bright. Within one to two visits, however, the patients might be making statements such as, "You are like all the rest," "You don't care," and so on. You will find that these patients are highly impulsive and self-destructive.

Patients with borderline personality disorder also demonstrate great affective instability and rapid shifts in mood and may become potentially suicidal without warning. They may show inappropriate and intense anger and may demonstrate recurrent suicidal threats or gestures, often in an attempt to manipulate others. These patients are highly uncertain of their self-image, goals, career choices, and values. Beneath the surface, these patients often experience chronic emptiness and intense boredom and ultimately admit to significant fear of being abandoned. In addition, they have self-hatred issues that they project onto others, becoming enraged over any hint of rejection, criticism, or abandonment. They also have major difficulties with compliance and a real potential for substance abuse. In attempting to deal with them, it is essential that your physician-patient relationship be structured from the outset, with clear limits on both behavioral and therapeutic expectations.

Borderline patients also have problems accepting boundaries and often attempt to set up inappropriate relationships or behave in a seductive manner. You must refrain from allowing them to call you by your first name and from calling them by theirs. They will attempt to take advantage of the relationship and try to turn it into a personal one. Physicians need to set and maintain clear limits on appropriate patient behavior, focus on specific goals, and refrain from treating the personality disorder. When behavior interferes with treatment, the behavior must be confronted; you may need to insist on psychological intervention, perhaps even as a condition of your ongoing treatment. When all this fails and no constructive changes are forthcoming, you may need to terminate treatment after giving proper notice and paying careful attention to due process.

Multidisciplinary centers have a decided advantage over single practitioners when dealing with patients who have comorbid psychiatric problems. The availability of psychiatric or psychological assistance can be easily coordinated, especially if the patient lives nearby. We suggest that you develop relationships with appropriate psychiatric or psychological colleagues to assist in the management of these complex and difficult patients. This can be particularly useful if these colleagues also have a background in and an understanding of the neurobiological basis of primary headache disorders.

Psychological Evaluation

Along with the initial detailed headache and medical history, physical and neurological examination, and laboratory tests, we include a psychophysiological assessment of all new patients. When psychological factors are clearly present, you might need to set up additional time to explore these more thoroughly via a clinical evaluation. It is important to have some understanding of the patient's history prior to the onset of their headaches.

The clinician should assess symptoms and difficulties associated with the pain, including changes and functional levels in all areas of living. Interpersonal, familial, vocational, and sexual areas should be investigated. Inquiries related to mood, sleep, appetite, and energy levels are relevant. Pay attention to the patient's current and past intake of medications and perhaps look for a history that might indicate abuse of alcohol or illicit drugs and prescription medications, particularly narcotics, barbiturates, sedative hypnotics, and benzodiazepines.

It may become clear that some patients are receiving medications from several prescribers and several pharmacies. It is important to establish at the outset that you will be the only prescriber of their headache medication and that only one pharmacy will be involved. Violations of these agreements may point to addictive behavior and require appropriate intervention before treatment can continue.

Narcotics, barbiturates, sedative hypnotism, and benzodiazepines may contribute on a biological basis to a patient's depression, may impair cognition, and may contribute to the pain through analgesic rebound. Patients who are overmedicated with β-blockers may also present with significant clinical symptoms of depression.

A formal mental status evaluation may be useful in terms of assessing affect, cognitive style, and more dramatic symptoms such as thought disorder or the presence of delusions and hallucinations. A family history that explores alcoholism, substance abuse, depressive disorders, anxiety disorders, psychiatric hospitalizations, and behavioral difficulties is relevant, too. If secondary gain is suspected, look for a history of physical symptoms in earlier life as an attention-getting form of behavior. Could the patient have "learned" a form of communication via physical illness?

It is essential to get a picture of the patient at work, at home, and at play. Past history might include inquiries about the patient's interpersonal style, particularly related to the experience and expression of strong emotions such as anger, rage, or resentment. To what extent does the patient value the approval of others over self-expression? The evaluation is designed to bring forth material that might reveal what, if any, psychiatric or psychological factors are involved in their current headache syndrome.

Psychological Testing

Psychological testing might include several instruments that are potentially useful in the evaluation of psychological and behavioral styles, such as the Minnesota Multiphasic Personality Inventory (MMPI), Beck Depression Inventory, Zung Self-Rating Depression Scale, the SCL-90, and a Holmes-Rahe Social Readjustment Rating Scale. These tools may all be useful and must be used in the context of the patient's disorder and clinical presentation. The MMPI is most useful in demonstrating somatization, personality styles, and overt psychiatric syndromes, although it cannot be readily interpreted by clinicians who lack experience in its use.

Kudrow and Sutkus (1979) demonstrated that the MMPI shows normal results in patients who have intermittent migraine. They found that patients who had more chronic headache showed evidence of more psychopathology on the MMPI. Those who have what they called "conversional" headache disorders demonstrated marked elevation of the first three scales, which involve hysteria, depression, and hypochondriasis. They also found this group of patients to be the most refractory to treatment and compared them to typical conversional patients with "la belle indifference." Other investigators point out that these elevations in the first three scales may in fact be caused by the greater intensity and chronicity of pain, which may masquerade as depressive symptomatology. Many patients, nonetheless, show a "somatic V," with elevation of the first and third scale and a much lower second scale, suggesting denial of depression and emphasis on physical symptomatology.

The Beck and Zung Scales focus primarily

on symptoms of depression and may also show abnormal results in patients with chronic pain. These scales are even more useful in a primary care setting and help to pick up and quantify clinical depression. The SCL-90 is a scale designed to detect evidence of clinically significant anxiety. We have found the Holmes-Rahe Social Readjustment Rating Scale useful in providing information about significant life changes that may have contributed to headache onset or changes in frequency of pain. These include factors such as death of a loved one, marriage, separation, divorce, and financial difficulties. Some studies have shown marked elevation of these parameters prior to the onset of headache.

Other tests may include achievement scales, locus of control assessments, assertiveness scales, Type-A behavior inventory, and marriage-family adjustment scales. Many of these can be administered, scored, and interpreted by computers. However, such data must not be accepted de novo and must be evaluated in the context of the individual patient. Finally, neuropsychological testing is indicated, particularly in cases of post-traumatic headache and post–head trauma syndrome in which clinical evaluation shows evidence of cognitive, intellectual, or memory deficits.

"The Headache Games"

Don Dalessio of San Diego described a number of headache games that patients play. The descriptions were based on James Groves' "Taking Care of the Hateful Patient." The following are a few of the classical games described by Dalessio. These presentations occur with regularity in chronic patients.

'It's my diet' game. "I know it is the food I am eating. I have given up most foods and all I eat now is scallions and broccoli with garlic powder. I never touch sugar and meat is bad for you. But I keep having headaches. Could I have some allergy tests?"

'It's my sinuses' game. "I have had my nose fixed, two Caldwell-Luc operations, and my turbinates removed, but I keep having sinus trouble. I can't breathe through my nose and the pain at the bridge of my nose is awful . . . if only I could get my nose and sinuses straightened out, everything would be fine."

'It's my TMJ' game. "I have been to three dentists and had complete caps. My bite has been reworked. I almost had my TM joints replaced. My teeth and gums burn all the time and my mouth is so sore I just can't stand it. Do you think it could be my dental fillings?"

'I need another test' game. "I am sure that there is something the matter, but the doctors can't find it. I have had three CT scans, three MRIs, and a bone scan, and they are all negative. Have you heard of magnetoencephalography? Should I have one of those? I will persist until I find an answer and I don't care how much it costs."

Dalessio goes on to describe a number of other similar games. We find that the common denominator running through almost all of these games is what we referred to in Chapter 7 as an external locus of control. In other words, these are patients who are looking for the magic bullet, the magic test, and the magic single answer to a very complex set of problems that is usually caused by a combination of the primary headache disorders. Here again, the relationship between the physician and patient is of paramount importance. It is the physician's job to educate as much as possible in order to prevent this endless search for "the answer." We have seen countless patients go to multiple doctors and have many tests, without satisfactory results.

Once organic pathology has been ruled out by reasonable history, examination, and testing, the most important goal is to help the patient move toward an internal locus of control and take responsibility for active participation in his or her recovery. It is certainly not unreasonable to rule out organic problems such as sinusitis or temporomandibular joint dysfunction if the clinical picture suggests these possibilities; however, ordering tests and evaluations just because everything else has been negative is usually a waste of time and money.

It is important to understand patients' resistance to accepting the concept of a primary headache disorder such as migraine, tension-type headache, or the clinical syndrome known as chronic daily headache. Perhaps the patient fears that if the problem is not related to a single demonstrable cause, then it must be psychological in the absence of biological markers and positive tests. At this point it is important to educate patients about the pathophysiology of primary headache disorders and to reassure them that indeed these disorders are "real" and physiological and not necessarily psychological in nature. However, in the patient who presents with multiple system involvement in the absence of organic findings, the diagnosis of a somatoform disorder should be considered and addressed.

Conclusion

The relationships between psychiatric factors, the human condition, and headache are indeed complex. It is important that professionals keep an open mind and believe that the patient's complaints are valid and that the pain is "real." Migraine and related disorders span a wide spectrum of frequencies, intensities, and durations. It has been observed that the more refractory patients who are totally unresponsive to outpatient therapies and are unable to stop their overuse of daily analgesics and ergots show a higher prevalence of medical and psychiatric comorbidity.

Most patients with occasional migraine and tension-type headache do well on their own and usually self-medicate appropriately with off-the-shelf nonprescription remedies. Moving down the scale, people will enter primary care offices as their headaches become more intense and more frequent and wind up in secondary care when their headaches become more chronic and refractory to treatment. Most of those who come to tertiary care headache centers have chronic daily headache associated with overuse syndromes and higher degrees of comorbidity. Patients who require inpatient treatment represent the most complex and difficult challenges, complicated by medication over-

use with multiple medical or psychiatric problems. For these patients, a coordinated, interdisciplinary effort is generally the best approach.

In their article in 1988 in *Scientific American* on "Plasticity in Brain Development," Chiye Aoiki and Phillip Siekevitz concluded as follows: "We are only beginning to understand how molecular events influence the structure of neurons and how these structural changes are translated into changes in brain function."

As we try to answer such questions, we hope to get closer to understanding how the external world comes to be mirrored in the microscopic structure of the brain. Ultimately, the answer will lead to a profound appreciation of how each individual person, in spite of being formed by inexorable genetic processes, is also the unique product of experience."

SUGGESTED READINGS

Alder CS, Alder SM, Packard RC: *Psychiatric Aspects of Headache.* Baltimore: Williams & Wilkins. 1987.

Alexander FG: *Psychosomatic Medicine: Its Principles and Applications.* New York: Norton. 1950.

American Psychiatric Association: *Diagnostical and Statistical Manual of Mental Disorders*, 3rd ed, revised. Washington DC: American Psychiatric Association. 1987. 3rd ed, 1987; 4th ed, 1994.

Bana DS, Graham JR, Spierings ELH: Headache patients as they see themselves. *Headache.* 1988;28:122–126.

Blanchard EB, Kirsch CA, Appelbaum KA, et al: Role of psychopathology in chronic headache: Cause or effect? *Headache.* 1989;29:295–301.

Blumer D: Chronic pain as a depressive disorder. *J Nerv Ment Dis.* 1982;170:381–406.

Breslau N, Davis GC: Migraine, major depression and panic disorder: A prospective epidemiologic study of young adults. *Cephalalgia.* 1992;12:85–90.

Breslau N, Davis GC, Schultz LR, et al: Migraine and major depression: A longitudinal study. *Headache.* 1994;34(7):387.

Couch JR, Ziegler DH, Hassanein RS: Evaluation of the relationship between migraine headache and depression. *Headache.* 1975;15:41.

Crisp AH, McGuinness B, Kalucy RS, et al: Some clinical, social and psychological characteristics of migraine subjects in the general population. *Postgrad Med J.* 1977;53:691.

Dalessio DJ, Silberstein SD: Clinical observations on headache. In Dalessio DJ, Silberstein SD, eds. *Wolff's Headache and Other Head Pain*, 6th ed. New York: Oxford University Press. 1993; 502.

Davis RA, Wetzel RD, Kashiwagi T, et al: Personality, depression and headache type. *Headache.* 1976; 16:246–251.

Diamond S: Depression and headache. *Headache.* 1983;23:122.

Eker Khour-Haddad S: Psychiatric consultation in a headache unit. *Headache.* 1984;24:322–326.

Engel G: Psychogenic pain and the pain-prone patient. *Am J Med.* 1959;26:899–918.

Friedman AP: Nature of headache. *Headache.* 1979; 19:163.

Friedman AP, Frazier SH: Preliminary observations of the psychiatric evaluation of treated chronic headache patients. *Res Clin Stud Headache* 1972;3:378.

Friedman AP, Storch TJC, Merritt HH: Migraine and tension headaches: A clinical study of two thousand cases. *Neurology.* 1954;4:773.

Friedman M: Type A behavior pattern: Some of its pathophysiological components. *Bull N Y Acad Med.* 1977;53:593.

Fromm-Reichman F: Contribution to the psychogenesis of migraine. *Psychoanal Rev.* 1937;24:26.

Glass DE: Tension headache and some psychiatric aspects. *Headache Q.* 1992;3:262–269.

Harrison RH: Psychological testing in headache: A review. *Headache.* 1975;14:177–185.

Kudrow L, Sutkus BJ: MMPI pattern specificity in primary headache disorders. *Headache.* 1979;19:18.

Lipowski ZJ: Somatization: The concept and its application. *Am J Psychiatry.* 1988;145:1358–1368.

Martin MJ: Tension headache: A psychiatric study. *Headache.* 1966;6:48.

Merikangas KR, Angst J, Isler H: Migraine and psychopathology: Results of the Zurich Cohort Study of Young Adults. *Arch Gen Psychiatry.* 1990;47:849.

Nappi G, Sandrini G, Granella F, et al: A new 5-HT$_2$ antagonist in the treatment of chronic headache with depression. A double-blind study vs. amitriptyline. *Headache.* 1990;30:439.

Ogren SO, Fuxe K, Agnati L: The importance of brain serotonergic receptor mechanisms for the action of antidepressant drugs. *Pharmacopsychiatry.* 1985; 18:209.

Packard RC: Life stress, personality factors, and reactions to headache. In Dalessio DJ, Silberstein SD, eds. *Wolff's Headache and Other Head Pain*, 6th ed. New York: Oxford University Press. 1993; 462.

Passachier H, Orlebeke JF: Personality and headache types: A controlled study. *Headache.* 1984;24:140–146.

Phillips C: Headache and personality. *J Psychosom Res.* 1976;20:535.

Roskies E: *Stress Management for the Healthy Type A: Theory and Practice.* New York: Guilford Press. 1987.

Selinsky H: Psychological study of the migrainous syndrome. *Bull N Y Acad Med.* 1939;15:757.

Sheftell FD: Chronic daily headache. *Neurology.* 1992;42(Suppl 2):32–36.

Sheftell FD: Psychological considerations in evaluation and treatment of headache disorders. In Rapoport AM, Sheftell FD, eds. *Headache: A Clinician's Guide to Diagnosis, Pathophysiology and Treatment Strategies.* Costa Mesa, CA: PMA Publishing Corp. 1993.

Sheftell FD, Silberstein SD, Rapoport AM, et al: Migraine and women: Diagnosis, pathophysiology and treatment. *Journal of Women's Health.* 1992;1:5–19.

Stenback A: Headache and life stress: A psychosomatic study of headache. *Acta Psychiatr Scand.* 1954; 92(Suppl):1–143.

Weeks R, Baskin S, Rapoport A, et al: A comparison of MMPI personality data and frontalis electromyographic readings in migraine and combination headache patients. *Headache.* 1983;23:75.

Wolff HG: Personality features and reactions of subjects with migraine. *Arch Neurol Psychiatry.* 1937;37:895.

Ziegler DK: Headache syndromes: Problems of definition. *Psychosomatics.* 1979;20(7):443.

Ziegler DK, Rhodes RJ, Hassanein RS: Association of psychological measurements of anxiety and depression with headache history in a non-clinic population. *Res Clin Stud Headache.* 1978;6:15.

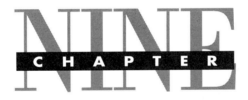

Emergency Room Evaluation and Treatment

Patients may require emergency room intervention when a headache syndrome becomes incapacitating. Incapacitating headaches may stem from a variety of causes, such as fever of unknown origin (FUO), intracranial hemorrhage, or other dramatic conditions. Some patients may be in the throes of the first significant headache of their lives or may be having the worst headache they have ever had. Both of these situations produce anxiety in addition to the obvious pain. Some "worst ever" headaches may represent a completely new type of headache or a new neurological condition. Such headaches may worsen progressively even though a recent medical evaluation may have revealed nothing. Other headaches draw to emergency rooms patients who have developed the "last straw" syndrome, a chronic and severe headache that has been unresponsive to treatment over a long period of time. The emergency room is where these patients go when they reach the end of their ability to cope with the headache.

Emergency Evaluation of Headache

Emergency room physicians should be concerned if patients who present to the emergency room have any of the problems just described. There is far less cause for concern when a diagnosis of migraine, acute severe tension-type headache, or cluster headache can be reasonably made. If, however, any of the red flags presented in Chapter 3 are present, it is vitally important to consider and rule out some more serious disease. Some of these causes for concern are:

1. *First* or *worst* headache of a patient's life
2. A headache that is *changing* in nature and severe
3. A headache that *worsens progressively* over days or weeks
4. A headache associated with *fever*, nausea, vomiting, and *stiff neck* or other *systemic illness*

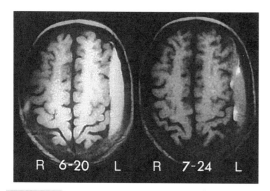

Figure 9–1

Emergency computed tomographic scan showing a dense subdural hematoma over the left cortex of the brain *(image on the left)*. One month later, the subdural hematoma is partially reabsorbed *(image on the right)*. (Courtesy of Dr. Rick Velaj, Radiology Department, Greenwich Hospital, Greenwich, CT.)

5. A headache with any *neurological symptoms* or *abnormal findings* on examination, such as hemisensory syndrome, hemiparesis, aphasia, focal visual problems; a worsening headache following recent *head trauma* could signal the need for further investigation

The diagnosis is made based on criteria covered in Chapter 2. In the emergency room, however, the history must usually be taken quickly. Keep in mind the red flags and inquire about past medical history such as any significant heart disease, metabolic or biochemical problems, exposure to toxic substances, or ingestion of certain headache-producing medications such as vasodilators, tetracycline, or vitamin A. A brief but complete medical and neurological examination must be conducted, with special attention to the heart and to the vascular system of the head and neck, especially in older patients. Sinus disease must be considered, and Lyme disease must be ruled out in areas of the United States where it is prevalent.

Emergency room diagnostic work-up must be decided on a case-by-case basis, as the appropriateness of various tests depends heavily on the situation. Patients with severe headache or neurological symptomatology after head trauma will need an emergency computed tomographic (CT) scan without contrast to rule out any evidence of intracranial hemorrhage (Fig. 9–1). A patient with a history of the first or worst headache

ever, or anyone with a history of changing headache also requires a CT scan. Contrast is not necessary when the scan is intended to search for bleeding or evidence of elevated intracranial pressure. It is often helpful to follow a non-contrast scan with a scan using intravenous contrast when evidence of tumor, aneurysm, or arteriovenous malformation is being sought. Although most headache specialists feel that magnetic resonance imaging (MRI) shows more detail and gives better views of special areas, such as the pituitary gland, the brain stem, and the cervicomedullary junction, MRI is more expensive, usually is not available on an emergency basis, and does not document acute hemorrhage as accurately as a CT scan. In most cases, a CT scan should suffice during the acute stage, followed by MRI at a later date if necessary.

Sinus x-rays may be helpful in patients with nasal and sinus pain, fever, or stuffed nose and postnasal drip in whom acute sinusitis is strongly suspected. If such x-rays reveal nothing abnormal, an emergency CT scan of the sinuses or an otolaryngological consultation with endoscopy may be indicated (Fig. 9–2).

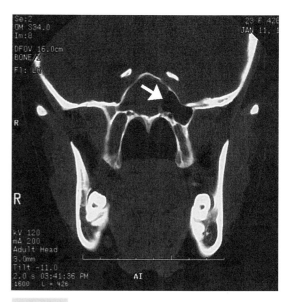

Figure 9–2

Coronal computed tomographic scan of the sinuses, demonstrating acute opacification of the right sphenoidal sinus *(arrow)*, which produced severe unilateral headache. (Courtesy of Dr. Rick Velaj, Radiology Department, Greenwich Hospital, Greenwich, CT.)

A lumbar puncture should be reserved for patients in whom rapid diagnosis is critically important, such as those with signs of meningitis. Lumbar puncture to rule out increased intracranial pressure should follow an emergency CT scan.

In some cases of mild subarachnoid hemorrhage, a CT scan may miss the bleeding; a carefully performed lumbar puncture in which a small amount of CSF is withdrawn via a thin (22 gauge or smaller) needle may clinch the diagnosis.

Most headache patients who come to the emergency room should have some screening blood work including measurement of electrolytes, a general chemistry profile, a complete blood count, and measurement of sedimentation rate. A Lyme titer should be performed when appropriate, but results are not usually available on an emergency basis.

The time to consider cerebral angiography is when an aneurysm or arteriovenous malformation is suspected in patients who have been diagnosed with a subarachnoid or intracerebral hemorrhage. Less frequently, the technique is used to look for cerebral arteritis. Doppler flow studies of the carotid artery can be conducted in older patients who have symptoms of transient ischemic attacks (TIAs) or signs of carotid artery disease (bruits over the carotid artery or diffuse evidence of arterial disease). Intracranial Doppler flow studies can be performed on older patients with signs or symptoms of cerebrovascular disease. MR angiography (MRA) can be a useful screening test for vascular disease, but false-negative results can occur.

Emergency Treatment of Headache

Treatment is dictated by specific diagnosis for patients with serious secondary causes of headache. Acute migraine, tension-type headache, and cluster headache can be treated with standard acute measures. Most patients with primary headache disorders present during a severe migraine attack or have migraine features superimposed on a severe attack of tension-type headache. We usually treat a severe migraine attack primarily with medications that we expect to abort the migraine process and only secondarily with pain medications. If, however, a patient comes into the emergency room having taken appropriate doses of abortive medication and is not doing well, he or she should receive potent analgesic and antiinflammatory medications for pain as well as antinausea or sedative medications, or both.

DIHYDROERGOTAMINE (D.H.E. 45)

Dihydroergotamine has been available for over 50 years and has been routinely used in the Greenwich Hospital Emergency Room for the past 15. Our standard method of administering this 5-HT$_1$ agonist is via a 1 mg intramuscular injection. Although it may not be absolutely necessary, we often give 50 mg IM of promethazine (Phenergan) and 4 mg IM of dexamethasone (Decadron), all in separate syringes. We find that this combination helps abort the migraine headache and relieves nausea and anxiety; patients rarely need follow-up doses for recurrent headache. Dihydroergotamine can also be given as a 1 mg subcutaneous dose, which is almost as effective, although it takes slightly longer to work.

Many emergency rooms start an intravenous drip of saline and give 10 mg of metoclopramide (Reglan) IV followed in 10 to 15 minutes by 0.5 to 1 mg of dihydroergotamine intravenously by slow push. Although this may produce faster relief, we consider it slightly more uncomfortable for patients and more risky, particularly for patients who will be sent home promptly. Furthermore, some patients become jittery or anxious after 10 mg of metoclopramide IV and may do slightly better when it is given by mouth or if promethazine is substituted. We use a similar protocol for patients who receive repeated intravenous doses of dihydroergotamine in the hospital (see Chapter 10). Other intravenous treatments include prochlorperazine (Compazine) and chlorpromazine (Thorazine). (See following paragraphs.)

SUMATRIPTAN (IMITREX)

Patients who have not taken ergotamine tartrate, dihydroergotamine, or other ergots within the previous 24 hours can be treated with 6 mg of sumatriptan subcutaneously, which usually relieves headache within 30 to 60 minutes; most side effects that occur (eg, paresthesias, flushing, nausea) are mild and transient. If patients develop chest tightness or pressure, an electrocardiogram should be performed to rule out coronary vasospasm while they are in the emergency room. If they respond successfully to Imitrex, patients should receive a prescription for an Imitrex starter pack with the self-injector or tablets and information on repeating the medication if the headache re-

curs (Fig. 9–3). Because there is a 30 to 50% recurrence rate within 24 hours, it is likely that the patient may need a second dose for recurrent headache. In addition, such patients should also be sent home with an antinausea medication as well as pain medication such as butorphanol nasal spray (Stadol NS) or Fiorinal with Codeine.

PROCHLORPERAZINE (COMPAZINE)

When patients cannot or will not take sumatriptan or dihydroergotamine, they can be given 10 mg of Compazine by slow IV push. This often has a dramatic effect on an acute migraine attack. Twenty-five mg of diphenhydramine (Benadryl) can be added

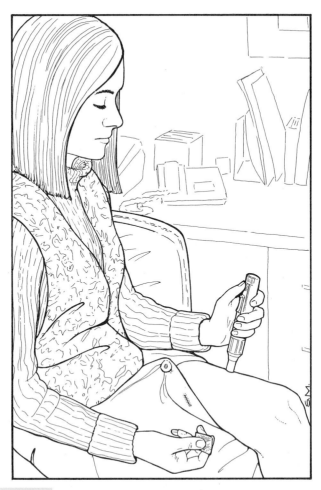

Figure 9–3

A patient self-injecting a subcutaneous dose of sumatriptan for the acute treatment of migraine.

to the intravenous solution to prevent dyskinesia.

CHLORPROMAZINE (THORAZINE)

Ten to 25 mg of Thorazine can be placed in 50 mL of normal saline and given intravenously over 20 to 30 minutes. It is best to give some normal saline and intravenously first because Thorazine can produce hypotension. Dizziness and drowsiness may occur. An alternative route of delivery is a 50 or 100 mg rectal suppository.

BENZODIAZEPINES

Benzodiazepines given intravenously, such as 10 mg of diazepam (Valium) or 2 mg or lorazepam (Ativan), can sometimes help with severe headache.

ANALGESICS

Some patients do well with a 60 mg intramuscular dose of ketorolac (Toradol), the only nonsteroidal anti-inflammatory medication that can be given parenterally. It may be helpful in up to 50% of acute migraine attacks, but it may cause gastrointestinal symptoms in highly sensitive patients or if overused. It can also cause nephrotoxicity.

Butorphanol nasal spray can be given as a 1 mg dose (one spray in one nostril), which can be repeated in 1 hour. In an emergency room setting, it may be given as a 2 mg dose intramuscularly. With lower abuse potential than other opiates, this opiate stimulates κ-immunoglobulin receptors rather than μ-immunoglobulin receptors and rapidly relieves pain without causing euphoria. Patients can be sent home with a bottle and instructed on its use. Side effects include drowsiness, dizziness, and dysphoria.

The standard treatment in many emergency rooms throughout the world is meperidine (Demerol) 50 to 100 mg IM mixed with promethazine (Phenergan) 50 mg IM or hydroxyzine (Vistaril) 50 mg IM. Other opiates can also be tried, such as 10 to 15 mg of morphine IM.

ANTIEMETICS

We treat most acute migraine attacks with antiemetics. We start with promethazine (Phenergan) 50 mg IM, by mouth or suppository, hydroxyzine (Vistaril) 50 mg IM or by mouth, prochlorperazine (Compazine) 5 or 10 mg by mouth, or trimethobenzamide (Tigan) 250 mg by mouth or 200 mg by suppository. Emetrol is a nonprescription carbohydrate liquid that has no side effects and may be taken in frequently repeated doses. The dose is 1 to 2 tablespoons every 30 minutes.

The newest antiemetic ondansetron (Zofran), 4 mg by mouth or approximately 8 mg IV, has proved extremely helpful in migraine patients with intractable vomiting. It may be difficult to find in emergency room formularies because it has been approved for the nausea and vomiting accompanying chemotherapy and is not usually given in the emergency room.

CORTICOSTEROIDS

We have found that when nothing else works to abort a migraine, 4 to 6 mg of dexamethasone (Decadron) orally, intramuscularly, or intravenously helps to decrease the discomfort of the headache over the next 2 to 4 hours. This dose can be repeated in 3 hours but should only be used once or twice per month to avoid complications.

Treatment of Acute Tension-Type Headache

By definition, an acute tension-type headache does not usually become severe and incapacitating and does not drive patients to the emergency room. However, if tension-type headache escalates and presents with migraine features, any of the measures described for migraine could be considered. In patients with severe headache but no evi-

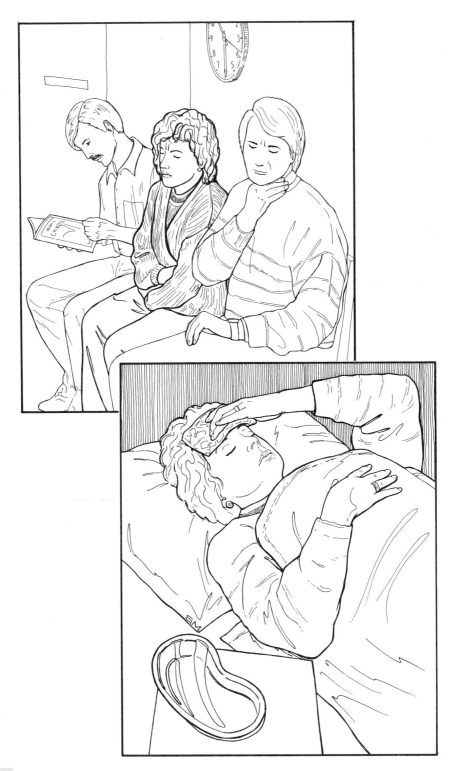

Figure 9–4

The wrong emergency room setting for headache *(top)* and the right emergency room setting for headache *(bottom)*. The wrong setting is busy, noisy, brightly lit, and nonprivate. The patient is sitting up and cold in the middle of much activity with bright lights. The correct setting is with the patient alone in a quiet, dimly lit room, lying on a stretcher covered by a blanket, with an emesis basin nearby and a cold compress on her forehead.

dence of a migraine process, benzodiazepines, analgesics, and possibly such muscle
relaxants as carisoprodol 350 mg (Soma) or
cyclobenzaprine 10 mg (Flexeril) may also
be helpful.

Cluster Headache

Given the average duration of cluster
headache of 45 to 90 minutes, by the time
patients with acute cluster headache arrive
in the emergency room, their headaches are
usually abating. Patient who present with
prolonged cluster attacks should be treated
initially with at least 7 L of oxygen per minute via a loose-fitting mask over the nose
and mouth while they are bent forward in
the sitting position breathing normally for
approximately 20 minutes. If this does not
break the headache, or if the headache keeps
returning, these patients can be given either
1 mg of dihydroergotamine intravenously or
subcutaneously, or 6 mg of sumatriptan subcutaneously. Some patients prefer an opiate,
and we would consider 1 mg of Stadol NS
(intranasally), 2 mg of Stadol IM, or 100 mg
of Demerol and 50 mg of Phenergan IM.
Sometimes we give patients our *triple shots*
consisting of D.H.E. 45 1 mg IM, Phenergan
50 mg IM, and Decadron 4 mg IM; this combination may be more effective than dihydroergotamine alone.

The Emergency Room Setting

Migraine patients do not look forward to
a visit to the emergency room. Such visits
are a major disruption for patients and their
families. Headache patients are often suspected of being drug-seeking and are usually
left in brightly lit, cold rooms while they
await evaluation. Emergency rooms can be
busy and chaotic. When possible, headache
patients should be placed in a darkened and
quiet area, should be allowed to lie down,
and should receive a blanket, cold pack, and
emesis basin while they await attention (Fig.
9–4). They always appreciate these considerations.

Follow-Up

When patients seek care in an emergency
medical department, they should be given
careful instructions on how and where to
obtain definitive follow-up headache care.
Some patients may be content to go back to
their own physicians, but others should be
referred to a knowledgeable neurologist,
headache specialist, or headache center. To
aid the educational process in the busy
emergency room, there should be literature
available that teaches the patient about
headache diagnosis and treatment and dis-
cusses follow-up care.

Although it is not common, some patients
have been effectively treated in an emergency room for the wrong reasons, and so
their headaches may reoccur several hours
or days later. We have seen patients with
subarachnoid hemorrhage, meningitis, and
brain tumor whose headaches were effectively treated in the emergency room but
who went on to develop more severe headache and the need for further definitive diagnostic testing and treatment. Always take
the emergency evaluation of a headache
problem seriously and proceed cautiously.

SUGGESTED READINGS

Belgrade MJ, Ling LJ, Scleevogt MG, et al: Comparison
of single-dose meperidine, butorphanol, and dihydroergotamine in the treatment of vascular headache.
Neurology. 1989;39:590–592.
Bell R, Montoya D, Shuaib A, et al: A comparative trial
of three agents in the treatment of acute migraine
headache. *Ann Emerg Med.* 1990;19:1079–1082.
Biousse V, D'Angletan JD, Touboui P, et al: Headache in
67 patients with extracranial internal carotid artery
dissection. *Cephalalgia.* 1991;11:232–233.
Callaham M, Raskin N: A controlled study of dihydroergotamine in the treatment of acute migraine
headache. *Headache.* 1086;2:168 171.
Day JW, Raskin NH: Thunderclap headache: Symptom
of unruptured cerebral aneurysm. *Lancet.* 1906;
29:1247–1248.
Dhopesh V, Anwar R, Herring C: A retrospective assessment of emergency department patients with complaint of headache. *Headache.* 1979;19:37–42.
Edmeads J: Emergency management of headache. *Headache.* 1988;28:675–679.
Gallagher RM: Emergency treatment of intractable migraine. *Headache.* 1986;26:74–75.
Harling DW, Peatfield RC, Van Hille PT, et al: Thunderclap headache: Is it migraine? *Cephalalgia.* 1989;
9:87–90.

Jones J, Sklar D, Dougherty J, et al: Randomized double-blind trial of intravenous prochlorperazine for the treatment of acute headache. *JAMA*. 1989;261:1174–1185.

Klapper JA, Stanton JS: The emergency treatment of acute migraine headache: A comparison of intravenous dihydroergotamine, dexamethasone, and placebo. *Cephalalgia*. 1991;11(Suppl 11):159–160.

Klapper JA, Stanton JS: Keterolac versus DHE and metoclopramide in the treatment of migraine headaches. *Headache*. 1991;31:523–524.

Lane PL, Ross R: Intravenous chlorpromazine: Preliminary results in acute migraine. *Headache*. 1985; 25:302–304.

Levine BD, Yoshimura K, Kobayashi T, et al: Dexamethasone in the treatment of acute mountain sickness. *N Engl J Med*. 1989;321:1707–1719.

Lew D, Southwick FS, Montgomery WW, et al: Sphenoid sinusitis: A review of 30 cases. *N Engl J Med*. 1983;19:1149-1154.

Olesen J, Aebelholt A, Veilis B: The Copenhagen acute headache clinic: Organization, patient material and treatment results. *Headache*. 1979;19:223–227.

Rapoport AM, Silberstein SD: Emergency treatment of headache. Neurology. 1992;42(Suppl 2):43–44.

Shesser R: Headache caused by serious illness: Evaluation in an emergency setting. *Postgrad Med J*. 1987; 81:117–125.

Silberstein SD: Evaluation and emergency treatment of headache. *Headache*. 1992; 32:396–407.

Wijdicks EFM, Kerkhoff H, Van Gijn J: Long-term follow-up of 71 patients with thunderclap headache mimicking subarachnoid hemorrhage. *Lancet*. 1988; 2:68–70.

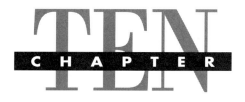

Inpatient Treatment of Primary Headache Disorders

Rapid changes in our health care system have led to an interesting dichotomy in the treatment of primary headache disorders. On the one hand, greater understanding of the pathophysiology of these conditions has resulted in improved treatment methods; on the other hand, access to appropriate care is becoming increasingly restricted. With a trend away from hospital admission towards outpatient care, many third-party payors strongly resist inpatient treatment for primary headache disorders. This reluctance notwithstanding, a small group of patients with primary headache disorders are debilitated and dysfunctional and often lead a "bed to couch" existence. They are dependent on opiates, benzodiazepines, barbiturates, and ergotamines and have become refractory to maximal outpatient intervention, even in the best of hands.

This chapter provides criteria for inpatient treatment and treatment protocols for this refractory group of headache patients. Figures 10–1 through 10–3 are forms that can help with hospital admission. Forms 1 and 2 (Figs. 10–1 and 10–2) help organize demographic information and admission criteria and suggest appropriate treatment

protocols that can be presented to third-party payors. Form 3, parts 1 and 2 (Fig. 10–3) is the temporary hospital admitting form that we use for temporary documentation until our dictated history, physical, diagnosis, and plan are on the chart.

Criteria for Inpatient Treatment

TRADITIONAL CRITERIA

The traditional criteria for inpatient evaluation and treatment of headache fall into two basic categories: *status migrainosis* in which severe, unrelenting migrainous headache associated with nausea and vomiting was persistent, lasted for several days, and was not manageable under outpatient care; and **presenting headache and concomitant neurological findings requiring a thorough work-up** to rule out structural pathology or other organic etiologies. The traditional approach to treatment usually included parenteral narcotics as needed or around the clock every 3 to 6 hours. Historically, little attention was paid to rebound phenomena and

HOSPITAL ADMISSION WORKSHEET

Date of Admission: _____ Inpatient Headache Unit

Diagnosis: _____ Time: _____

SEX: ___ M ___ F RACE: _____

PATIENT NAME: _____ Religion: _____

Birthdate: _____ Social Security Number: _____

Address-Street: _____

City: _____ State: _____ Zip: _____

Home telephone: _____ Work: _____

PERSON RESPONSIBLE FOR BILL: _____

RELATIONSHIP TO PATIENT: _____

PERSON'S EMPLOYER: _____

Birthdate: _____ Social Security Number: _____

Address-Street: _____

City: _____ State: _____ Zip: _____

Telephone: _____ Work: _____

PATIENT'S EMPLOYER: _____ Occup: _____

Address-Street: _____

City: _____ State: _____ Zip: _____

Telephone: _____ Work: _____

PERSON TO NOTIFY IN AN EMERGENCY: _____

RELATIONSHIP TO PATIENT: _____

Address-Street: _____

City: _____ State: _____ Zip: _____

Telephone: _____ Work: _____

INSURANCE INFORMATION: Insurance Forms Received: _____

Insurance Co: _____

Address-Street: _____

City: _____ State: _____ Zip: _____

I.D. #: _____ GROUP #: _____

Telephone: _____

PRECERTIFICATION:

Date Called: _____ Contact Person: _____

Status: _____

© The New England Center for Headache

Figure 10–1

Pre-admission precertification form used to organize the patient's demographic data for presentation to a third-party payor.

medication overuse, as is sometimes still true today.

Over the years, patients have been referred to us who were recently in the hospital where they received meperidine (Demerol) 100 mg every 3 hours for 4 or more days. Although opiates may help to stave off the pain for several hours, they do not address the underlying pathophysiology of headache and may easily produce dependency. Many of these patients were discharged after several hospital days without permanent headache control and a formalized discharge plan with recommendations for ongoing therapy having been established. Admission and subsequent discharge of such patients generally results in wasted efforts on the part of physicians and nurses, unnecessary costs to the health care system, and little contribution toward ongoing relief.

CURRENT CRITERIA

We suggest that the following criteria be used in evaluating patients for inpatient treatment:

1. Intractable severe headache that is unresponsive to appropriate outpatient treatment.
2. Severe headache that significantly interferes with
   a) quality of life.
   b) the ability to carry out the functions of daily living at work, home, and play.
3. Severe headache with increasing dependence on
   a) opiates.
   b) barbiturate-containing analgesics.
   c) ergotamine tartrate.
   d) benzodiazepines and sedative hypnotics.
   e) nonprescription medications, including salicylates, acetaminophen, and nonsteroidal anti-inflammatory agents, with toxicity symptoms including tinnitus, evidence of renal impairment (eg, elevated blood urea nitrogen and creatinine levels), gastrointestinal

HOSPITAL PRE-ADMISSION CERTIFICATION SHEET
GREENWICH HOSPITAL IN-PATIENT HEADACHE PROGRAM

NAME: _____   DATE: _____

   D.O.B. _____ / _____ / _____   Physician:

   SS # _____ / _____ / _____   AR _____

                             FS _____

                             DM _____

                             Other _____

NAME OF INSURED: _____

PRIMARY INSURANCE: _____

   D.O.B. _____ / _____ / _____   SS # _____ / _____ / _____

DIAGNOSIS: REASON FOR ADMISSION:

____ Post Traumatic Headache   ____ Intractable Migraine Headache

____ Intractable Migraine   ____ Intractable Cluster Headache

____ Migraine Without Aura   ____ Unresponsive to Outpatient Rx

____ Migraine With Aura   ____ Parenteral Rehydration Required

____ Tension-Type Headache   ____ Increasing Use/or Dependence on Pain Medication

____ Analgesic Rebound Headache   ____ Associated Depression/Anxiety

____ Ergotamine Rebound Headache   ____ Comorbid Medical Problems:

____ Cluster Headache   _____   _____   _____

____ Other   _____   _____   _____

Onset: _____

                       (____ Overuse of Opiates: _____   Qty: _____

Duration of Worsening: _____   (____ Overuse of Analgesics: _____   Qty: _____

                       (____ Overuse of Barbiturates: _____   Qty: _____

Symptoms: N _____V _____ A _____ D _____   Dizzy _____   Sono _____   Photo _____

         Worse with Activity _____ Extent of Disability _____

Previous Medications: _____   _____   _____

                         _____   _____   _____

                         _____   _____   _____

                         _____   _____   _____

Current Medications: _____   _____   _____

                         _____

Medications & Quantities in the Week prior to Admission:

_____   _____   _____   _____

Figure 10–2

Form used to record the patient's admission criteria, clinical data, and possible treatment plan for presentation to a third-party payor.

Illustration continued on following page

Previous Testing: *Abnormal Results:* _____

CT Head	Date: _____	CT Cervical Spine	Date: _____
Contrast Y ___ N ___		MRI Cervical Spine	Date: _____
MRI Head	Date: _____	EKG	Date: _____
EEG	Date: _____	Thyroid	Date: _____
LP	Date: _____	Lyme	Date: _____
Other/Date: _____		Other	Date: _____

Treatment Plan:

_____ IV DHE for 5 days, IV Decadron for 2 days, or other _____

_____ Detoxification   1-Opiates   2-Barbiturates   3-Analgesics   4-Ergots   _____ Other

_____ Oral Medications _____   _____   _____   _____   _____

_____ Evaluation and Treatment by all Members of the Headache Treatment Team.

_____ Other _____

_____

©The New England Center for Headache

Figure 10–2

Continued

bleeding, evidence of hepatotoxicity, and overuse syndromes. These toxic sequelae represent hidden costs to the health care system. Many headache patients have been admitted for gastrointestinal hemorrhage, ulcers, and gastritis secondary to overuse of aspirin and nonsteroidal anti-inflammatory agents, but are not usually classified as an admission due to headache.

4. The probability of severe rebound headache upon withdrawal of current medications. If patients are unable to adhere to outpatient protocols to reduce the use of offending agents that cause rebound and dependence, hospital admission for more aggressive therapies should be considered.

5. Severe headache with increasing frequency of costly emergency room visits. We have seen many patients who are in the emergency room once or twice per week for parenteral opiate therapy. These patients are often accused of drug-seeking behavior when such is usually not the case. Emergency room visits are disruptive to patients and their families, and although they are at times necessary, it is usually possible to avoid them with appropriate use of effective abortive agents after hospitalization.

6. Severe headache associated with comorbid medical problems that complicate outpatient interventions and require close monitoring and treatment. These include coronary artery disease, uncontrolled hypertension, ulcer disease, renal and hepatic dysfunction, and asthma.

7. Severe headache with comorbid psychiatric problems such as depression with hopelessness, sleeplessness, and severe anxiety disorder.

8. Severe headache associated with protracted nausea, vomiting, and dehydration that necessitate intravenous fluid replacement.

9. Intractable cluster headache with no response to appropriate outpatient therapy.

PRACTICAL CONSIDERATIONS REGARDING PRE-CERTIFICATION

Figure 10-2 provides a format for recording the salient features that justify inpatient treatment. This form can be used as a template for discussion with appropriate third-party payor review personnel. We find

GREENWICH HOSPITAL TEMPORARY ADMISSION SHEET (SIDE 1)

Patient Stamp

Side 1 must be completed for all patients

I. Reason for Admission:
   Chief complaints and brief pertinent note

II. Other Known Acute or Chronic Problems (which might affect care)—include medications and allergies:

III. Impression:

IV. Plan (Note appropriate completed studies):

V. Personal, Past, Social and Family History:
   [   ] on chart-reviewed and up to date
   [   ] Dictated—Date _____   Date Dictated: _____

VI. Permanent Admitting Note and Physical Examination
   Must be dictated within 24 hours of admission.

VII. Comments:

(see reverse side for Physical Exam)

Figure 10–3

Form used for temporary documentation of the patient's admitting history and physical examination, used until the relevant dictated information has been transferred to the patient's chart. (Courtesy of Greenwich Hospital.)

Illustration continued on following page

that the medical personnel at the institutions that provide health coverage require education about primary headache disorders in general as well as about the rationale for inpatient therapy. Citing literature and relevant outcome data that support these kinds of interventions helps to strengthen the case for in-hospital treatment.

Sample Model

Of the many tertiary care outpatient centers within the United States, only a few have dedicated headache inpatient units at affiliated hospitals. Hospital admissions may come about as a result of the initial outpatient evaluation. For example, at The New England Center for Headache, some patients who are referred to us clearly need inpatient intervention and have often received appropriate outpatient care without improvement. Other patients require admission only after reasonable attempts at outpatient therapy at our Center. Some patients become refractory to outpatient therapy.

Once the criteria for hospital admission have been met, patients are referred to a staff

GREENWICH HOSPITAL TEMPORARY ADMISSION SHEET (SIDE 2)

All items <u>must</u> be covered in the permanent admitting note which is to be dictated within 24 hours of admission:

Key: √ = Examined and essentially normal.   0 = None or Absent
NE = Not Examined

Vital Signs: T _____ P _____ R _____ B/P _____

General Appearance: _____

_____

HEENT: _____

Heart: _____ Chest: _____ Breasts: _____

Lungs: _____ Genitalia: M _____ F _____

Abdomen: _____

Skin: _____ Rectal: _____

Extremities: _____ Pelvic: _____

Neurological: _____

Other pertinent physical findings: _____

_____

_____

_____

_____

FOR HOUSE STAFF: Admission Lab Studies

Hct: _____   EKG:
Rhythm: _____
WBC: _____
Rate: _____
Diff: _____
Axis: _____
Urine Analysis: _____
Interpretation: _____
Lytes: _____
_____
ABGs: _____
Chest x-ray: _____
Other: _____

_____   _____
Date   M.D. Signature

Figure 10–3

Continued

member who is specifically responsible for hospital liaison and is dedicated to working with third parties to secure admission pre-certification. This staff member then coordinates all details of the patient's admission to the headache unit (Fig. 10–4). Patients and their families are educated as to the need for admission and are told what to expect in the hospital; goals and specifics of treatment are reviewed. Prior to admission, the hospital staff receives information relating to diagnoses and comorbid medical problems, along with the initial treatment plan orders.

The New England Center for Headache's outpatient interdisciplinary team approach is duplicated at the inpatient headache unit. Comprehensive medical and headache history as well as physical and neurological examinations are reviewed and dictated from the office as an admitting note. Laboratory tests are ordered as necessary, and cardiograms are done either prior to or on the day of admission because vasoactive medi-

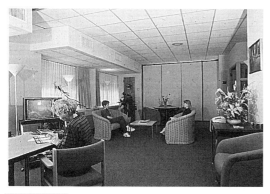

Figure 10-4

The Greenwich Hospital Inpatient Headache Unit, showing the eating and living area where patients can sit comfortably in their own clothes, attend group sessions, relax, eat, or exercise. (Courtesy of Hank Shull Photography.)

cations are likely to be used aggressively. By the time most patients reach the hospital, major testing such as neuroimaging has usually been completed.

The interdisciplinary evaluation at the hospital is summarized as follows:

Nursing Evaluation

The patient is oriented to the unit and undergoes a full nursing assessment. Nurses are involved in monitoring the administration of intravenous medications, patients' day-to-day progress, and interactions on the unit. Nurses are integrally involved in running orientation, relaxation, and relapse prevention groups and in discharge planning in general.

Physician Admission Assessment

An intervening history is taken, complete physical examination is performed by the admitting physician, and the treatment plan is updated and presented to the patient and discussed with the nursing staff.

Psychological/Behavioral Assessment

These assessments are performed by PhD clinical psychologists who also serve as clinical program directors of the unit. They review the patient's history, psychological status, and physiological profile and make recommendations for behavioral and other interventions.

Social Work Evaluation

The unit social worker meets with the family and significant others on the day of admission and does an assessment of the family and the effect of headache on the patient and the family and makes suggestions for discharge planning.

Physical Therapy Evaluation

Patients are assessed by physical therapists who focus on symptoms referable to the neck and jaw. Physical therapy on our unit consists mostly of educating and retraining patients with postural corrections and exercises. Physical therapy is geared toward self-help methods rather than more traditional applications of modalities, although these certainly are used when indicated.

Exercise and Conditioning Evaluation and Education

Patients have four sessions of education in the value of conditioning; they have individual assessments by an exercise physiologist, and some patients begin to exercise daily on equipment available in the unit.

Nutritional Assessment

The nutritionist assigned to the unit reviews the patients' nutritional status, educates them about our migraine elimination diet and low fat diets, and makes other appropriate suggestions regarding meal planning and caffeine intake.

Pharmacist Evaluation and Education

The hospital pharmacist plays an integral role on the unit. He assesses each patient's medication history and remains involved in ongoing evaluation of pharmacotherapy with the following in mind: patient history, comorbid medical problems, possible side effects, adverse reactions, rebound syndromes and drug-drug interactions.

Occupational Therapy Evaluation

The occupational therapist reviews patients' vocational and leisure time activities and makes concrete suggestions, specifically with respect to time management and quality time for oneself.

Hospital Chaplain Group

The hospital chaplain is involved with the team and may co-lead groups with other members of the team. We find that many of our patients appreciate attention to the spiritual aspects of their lives.

Administration

The headache unit to which we admit patients is co-administered by a physician medical director and a PhD clinical director. They coordinate and integrate the interdisciplinary team approach that we believe is essential to the treatment of these most refractory headache patients.

Outcome Studies

At this point, we are not aware of any outcome studies that compare these interdisciplinary approaches with the routine admission of refractory patients for pharmacological therapy alone. A sufficient number of reports in the literature, however, support improved outcome when pharmacological and nonpharmacological measures are integrated as detailed previously. Our own studies show that on discharge, 80% of our patients have significantly improved and that 6 months later, that figure is 75%.

Inpatient Treatment Strategies

PHARMACOLOGICAL THERAPY

The mainstay of pharmacological therapy for refractory patients with primary head-

ache disorders is the use of intravenous dihydroergotamine (D.H.E. 45) (Fig. 10–5). The rationale for its use is based on its mechanisms of action and on outcome studies. D.H.E. 45 is a potent serotonin agonist that inhibits neurogenic inflammation in the meninges and has a role in the modulation of central serotonergic pain mechanisms. Dihydroergotamine has binding cites in the midbrain dorsal raphe nucleus, the spinal cord dorsal horn, and the trigeminal nucleus caudalis, all integrally involved with head pain.

The fact that D.H.E. 45 has both peripheral and central actions may give it a decided advantage over agents that have peripheral actions alone in the treatment of refractory headache disorders. Raskin, in his landmark publication of 1986, outlines the treatment protocols for the use of intravenous D.H.E. 45 for refractory patients. These protocols have been modified by others throughout the country, but most are based on his initial prototype. Raskin found that the average length of hospital stay for headache patients treated with dihydroergotamine was shorter and the demonstrated improvement over the long term was greater than that seen in patients treated traditionally with protocols of narcotics or benzodiazepines.

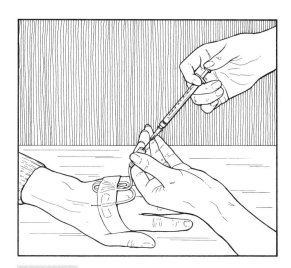

Figure 10–5

Patient receiving repetitive intravenous dihydroergotamine (D.H.E. 45) via a heparin lock for the treatment of chronic daily headache with analgesic rebound.

Long-term outcome studies by Silberstein and Saper and our group have shown decreased debilitation, decreased use of abortive medication, decreased visits to the emergency room, and increased functional capacity in patients treated with repetitive intravenous D.H.E. 45 in an inpatient, interdisciplinary setting over a 7- to 10-day period.

Medication Protocols

We generally start patients on an intravenous dose of 0.25 mg of D.H.E. 45 and titrate to between 0.5 and 1 mg, depending on side effects and response to therapy. If patients do not respond within the first 24 hours to a starting dose, we raise the dose gradually to 1 mg. Our 5-day protocol specifies that patients receive dihydroergotamine three times daily for the first 2 or 3 days, with gradual reduction over the next 2 days. The dihydroergotamine is administered through a heparin lock and is delivered by barbotage or a push-pull method. A small amount is injected, then some blood is pulled back into the syringe, and then advanced again slowly over a 3- to 5-minute period (see Fig. 10–5). We may use any one of a number of oral antiemetics 30 minutes prior to dihydroergotamine administration; these include promethazine (Phenergan) at 25 to 50 mg, metoclopramide (Reglan) at 5 or 10 mg, and prochlorperazine (Compazine) at 10 to 25 mg. When nausea or vomiting is protracted and unresponsive to these antiemetics, we may use 4 mg of ondansetron (Zofran).

When patients do not respond well to oral antiemetic medications we give appropriate doses of intramuscular, rectal, or intravenous therapy; we find that the nonprescription antiemetic Emetrol, in 1- to 2-tablespoon doses, may be helpful as well. Metoclopramide may produce agitation and extrapyramidal effects, particularly akathisia, especially when given intravenously. Patients may experience this phenomenon as restlessness, anxiety, or insomnia. We tend to avoid metoclopramide in patients who have underlying anxiety disorders. If patients are not responding to maximal doses of intravenous D.H.E. 45, we may add a steroid, usually dexamethasone (Decadron) at a dose of 4 mg IV twice daily the first day and once daily on the second day. Occasionally we extend the treatment to 5 days. Hydrocortisone at a dose of 100 mg IV may also be used in the same manner.

Side Effects of D.H.E. 45

Nausea and muscle or abdominal cramps are the most common side effects of IV D.H.E. 45. Other side effects include diarrhea, head tightness, a sensation of warmth, chest pain, light-headedness, vomiting, transient increase in headache, potential supraventricular tachycardia when co-administered with nortriptyline (two cases reported by Raskin), and transient mild elevation of blood pressure. Dihydroergotamine is a more potent venoconstrictor than an arterial constrictor. The management of these side effects includes appropriate titration of antiemetics, dose reduction of dihydroergotamine, and reassurance that these side effects are transient and will dissipate as the dose is reduced.

Contraindications to Dihydroergotamine Therapy

Contraindications include peripheral vascular disease, coronary artery disease, Prinzmetal's angina, impaired renal or hepatic function, vasospastic disease, pregnancy, stroke, transient ischemic attack, hypersensitivity to ergotamine tartrate, and acute thrombophlebitis. Patients who are hypersensitive to ergotamine tartrate do not usually experience the same effects with dihydroergotamine. However, we are cautious and administer only a very small dose (0.1 mg) intravenously the first time dihydroergotamine is used in this situation.

Treatment of Overuse Syndromes (Including Dependency)

Treatment of overuse syndromes with abortive and symptomatic medications is an essential and crucial part of inpatient therapy. Many patients who have received IV D.H.E. 45 before coming to see us also received concomitant intramuscular injections of meperidine or intravenous diazepam. It has been our experience and that of others that the co-administration of these agents detracts from the potential efficacy of repetitive IV D.H.E. 45.

We can divide the treatment of overuse syndromes into several categories, delineated by type of medication overused, including nonprescription medications, opiates, barbiturates, ergotamine tartrate, and benzodiazepines.

NONPRESCRIPTION MEDICATION

Nonprescription medication may be abruptly discontinued, and rebound pain will generally be alleviated quite adequately by intravenous D.H.E. 45. However, one should be aware of the patient's total caffeine intake in nonprescription medication and caffeine-containing beverages. When caffeine intake is 300 mg or greater per day we taper that intake by 100 mg every other day. When caffeine intake is 500 mg or greater per day we taper it by 100 mg every 5 days. If caffeine dependency is overlooked, many patients will experience a marked increase in their headaches and a variety of other symptoms secondary to abrupt withdrawal from caffeine.

OPIATES

We generally taper opiates using the offending agent itself. We taper Tylenol with codeine by 30 mg of codeine every 24 hours or more rapidly as tolerated. As a general rule of thumb, since most patients are overusing oral opiates, withdrawal can be accomplished by decreasing the daily dose by one or two tablets of whatever substance they are taking. Concomitant use of clonidine at a dose of 0.05 mg twice or three times daily may aid in achieving a symptom-free withdrawal. Once the opiate is discontinued, clonidine should be continued

for another 72 hours; after that period, it, too, should be tapered over a period of 72 hours.

As an alternative to oral clonidine, the Catapres-TTS-1 or TTS-2 patches can be used. These patches provide a constant level of clonidine for 7 days, equivalent to 0.1 or 0.2 mg per day. The clinician should be aware that clonidine and amitriptyline may block each other's effect.

BARBITURATES

Abrupt withdrawal from barbiturates or benzodiazepines can provoke uncomfortable symptoms and possibly seizures. We generally replace the short-acting butalbital with long-acting phenobarbital. The conversion ratio is 30 mg of phenobarbital per 100 mg of butalbital. The phenobarbital is given in divided doses throughout the day and tapered by 15 to 30 mg every 24 to 48 hours, accompanied by close monitoring of vital signs, neurological symptoms, and anxiety, which suggests that withdrawal may be too rapid. High doses of divalproex sodium (Depakote) should be avoided when phenobarbital is used, as this agent may potentiate the actions of phenobarbital.

ERGOTAMINE TARTRATE

Because IV dihydroergotamine works very well to minimize any withdrawal effects, ergotamine tartrate can be abruptly discontinued. Clonidine may be useful in this case, too, in decreasing withdrawal symptoms. Our experience and most outcome studies show that patients who are experiencing rebound headache from single agent ergotamine tartrate do very well with the IV D.H.E. 45 protocol and are often free of headache in one week.

BENZODIAZEPINES

Benzodiazepines need to be tapered very slowly. We generally taper diazepam (Valium) 2.5 mg per week and alprazolam

(Xanax) 0.5 mg per week. Clonidine has been mentioned in the literature as being potentially helpful. The psychiatric literature suggests that the use of anticonvulsants such as carbamazepine may decrease withdrawal time.

Treatment of Breakthrough Headaches in the Hospital

This is a very important aspect of inpatient treatment. We do everything possible to discourage the use of opiates except when they are being used on a regular withdrawal schedule. We do not use opiates as nighttime medication, as they may hamper the potential effectiveness of intravenous dihydroergotamine. We discourage the use of prn medication for mild headaches and suggest that patients use the variety of nonpharmacological measures available to them. These measures include the application of ice or heat, depending upon which is more effective, physical therapy exercises, relaxation, biofeedback techniques, and support from the nursing staff or patient peers on the unit.

If we must advance to pharmacological measures, we start conservatively with the milder oral medications such as isometheptene mucate in the form of Midrin, two capsules stat repeated in 1 hour if needed. Next we try one of several nonsteroidal agents such as meclofenamate (Meclomen) at a dose of 100 to 200 mg by mouth, repeated in 1 to 2 hours if necessary, or naproxen sodium (Anaprox) at a dose of 550 mg with a similar repeat schedule.

If we must progress to the next level of intervention, we give intramuscular hydroxyzine (Vistaril) 50 mg or ketorolac (Toradol) 30 to 60 mg as rescue therapy.

Finally, if we must resort to intravenous intervention, we generally use chlorpromazine (Thorazine), placing 10 mg in 50 mL of normal saline and administering it over 30 minutes with the patient lying in bed. This can be repeated if the patient is still awake or if the headache intensity is unchanged. It is important to monitor vital signs during administration and to watch for potential orthostasis. If the starting blood pressure is low, it may be wise to inject 250 mL of normal saline before the chlorpromazine.

All of these pharmacological techniques are carried out in the context of an interdisciplinary team approach. Patients are assessed and treated individually by various members of the team. They attend groups run by nurses, social workers, psychologists, pharmacists, occupational and physical therapists, and the hospital chaplain, all addressing a variety of aspects of headache management. Patients are thoroughly educated as to the appropriate use of medication on an as-needed basis and to nonpharmacological techniques, all geared to prevent relapse due to medication overuse, rebound, or dependency phenomena.

Discharge Planning

Discharge planning actually starts on the first hospital day. All the techniques used in the inpatient program are similar to those employed in Alcoholics Anonymous programs, such as relapse prevention training. Patients receive specific guidelines, their use of calendars is reinforced, and they learn a step-wise intervention plan for their most severe headaches. They may be given first-line, second-line, and third-line therapies to abort the headache and prevent emergency room visits. A discharge group meeting that reinforces all of these measures is run on the day prior to discharge. We encourage patients to use nonpharmacological approaches for the relief of mild and moderate headaches and to move on to pharmacological interventions for severe or incapacitating headaches.

The family participates in a discharge conference on the day of discharge, and their concerns are addressed. It is helpful to advise family members not to ask patients on a daily basis, "How is your headache today?" Rather, patients are instructed to communicate their level of pain and their plan of action. Patients are generally seen in follow-up 1 to 2 weeks after discharge. For those who come from far away, we monitor their progress through the use of headache calendars. We work closely with local physicians and attempt to monitor patients via phone contact and by fax. When absolutely necessary, long distance patients come in for revisits once or twice per year.

Conclusion

In summary, inpatient intervention is reserved for approximately 10 to 15% of our patients, those who remain refractory to even the most aggressive outpatient approaches. Specific criteria determine the need for inpatient therapy. One must argue long and convincingly with third- and fourth-party payors for precertification and approval of an appropriate number of days of hospital stay. The usual length of stay on our unit is 6 to 9 full days. In cases of pronounced dependency, longer stays may be necessary. When substance abuse problems are clearly evident, we work closely with the alcohol and drug recovery unit at Greenwich Hospital. Patients may attend their group meetings and receive appropriate referrals upon discharge.

Our own outcome data and that of other investigators show that hospital treatment for refractory headache is a very cost-effective intervention in this difficult-to-treat population. Such treatment produces long-term reductions in the number of emergency room visits, sustained decreases in use of opiates and other analgesics, improved functional status, and overall improvement in quality of life. Our long-term (6-month) sustained improvement rate is 75% of hospitalized patients.

SUGGESTED READINGS

Bakris GL, Cross PD, Hammarsten JE: The use of clonidine for management of opiate abstinence in a chronic pain patient. *Mayo Clin Proc.* 1982;57:657.

Bonica JJ: Multidisciplinary/interdisciplinary pain programs. In Bonica JJ, ed. *The Management of Pain,* vol 1. Philadelphia: Lea & Febiger. 1990.

Diamond S: Inpatient treatment of headache. *Clin J Pain.* 1989;5:101–103.

Diamond S, Freitag FG, Maliszewski M: Inpatient treatment of headache: Long-term results. *Headache.* 1986;2:189–198.

Klapper JA: Denial of hospitalization by insurers for inpatient treatment of medication rebound headaches. *Headache.* 1994;34:601–602.

Lake AE, Saper JR, Madden SF, et al: Comprehensive inpatient treatment for intractable migraine: A prospective long-term outcome study. *Headache.* 1993; 33:55–62.

Rapoport AM, Weeks RE, Baskin SM, Sheftell FD: Inpatient headache treatment: Analysis of outcome post-discharge. *Neurology.* 1995;45(Suppl 4):A379.

Rapoport AM, Weeks RE, Sheftell FD, et al: Analgesic rebound headache: Theoretical and practical implications. *Cephalalgia.* 1989;5(supp 3):448–450.

Raskin NH: Repetitive intravenous dihydroergotamine as therapy for intractable migraine. *Neurology.* 1986; 36:995–997.

Silberstein SD, Silberstein JR: Analgesic/ergotamine rebound headache: Prognosis following detoxification and treatment with repetitive IV DHE. *Headache.* 1992;32:352.

Index

Note: Page numbers in *italics* refer to illustrations; page numbers followed by t refer to tables.